1.15.79

# Peter Lupus' Guide to Radiant Health and Beauty:

# Mission Possible for Women

*Peter Lupus*

*Samuel Homola, D.C.*

A Word from Lee Meriwether
A Foreword—Frank S. Caprio, M.D.

PARKER PUBLISHING COMPANY

# Peter Lupus' Guide to Radiant Health and Beauty:

## Mission Possible for Women

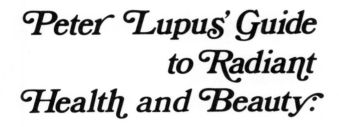

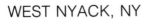

WEST NYACK, NY

*Peter Lupus' Guide to*
*Radiant Health and Beauty:*
*Mission Possible for Women*
by Peter Lupus and Samuel Homola, D.C.

© 1978 *by*

PARKER PUBLISHING COMPANY, INC.

West Nyack, NY

Library of Congress Cataloging in Publication Data

Lupus, Peter
  Peter Lupus' guide to radiant health and beauty.

  Includes index.
    1. Women—Health and hygiene.  2. Beauty, Personal.
I. Homola, Samuel, joint author.  II. Title.  III. Ti-
tle: Guide to radiant health and beauty.
RA778.L95        613'.04244        77-16668
ISBN 0-13-661884-7

Printed in the United States of America

*Dedicated to women everywhere,*
*who are all beautiful in some special way.*

2037151

*Acknowledgments*

Line drawings by Bibiana Neal.
Photographs by Tom Needham and Kenny Studer.

Books by Samuel Homola:

*Bonesetting, Chiropractic, and Cultism*
*Backache: Home Treatment and Prevention*
*A Chiropractor's Treasury of Health Secrets*
*La Salud y Sus Secretos*
*Muscle Training for Athletes*
*Secrets of Naturally Youthful Health and Vitality*
*Doctor Homola's Natural Health Remedies*
*Doctor Homola's Life-Extender Health Guide*
*Doctor Homola's Fat-Disintegrator Diet*

# About the Authors

The combined knowledge and experience of Dr. Samuel Homola and Peter Lupus, the authors of this book, provide special, *original* material that cannot be duplicated in any other book.

Dr. Homola is the author of more than 300 articles and 10 books in the field of health. He has had 20 years of experience in handling the health problems of patients.

Peter Lupus, best known for his role in the television series "Mission: Impossible," is a recognized health-and-exercise authority as well as an internationally known movie and television star. His association with stars and models all over the world has revealed to him the secrets of physically beautiful people. His own outstanding physical appearance has earned him such titles as "Mr. Indiana," "Mr. International Health," and *Playgirl* magazine's "Man of the Year" award.

In addition to acting and writing, Peter Lupus has been serving as a professional consultant to the nation's top health spas and figure salons for over 15 years. A frequent guest on such nationally televised shows as "The Merv Griffin Show" and Dinah Shore's "Dinah's Place," his views on exercise and nutrition have generated a great demand for his guidance in personal health programs.

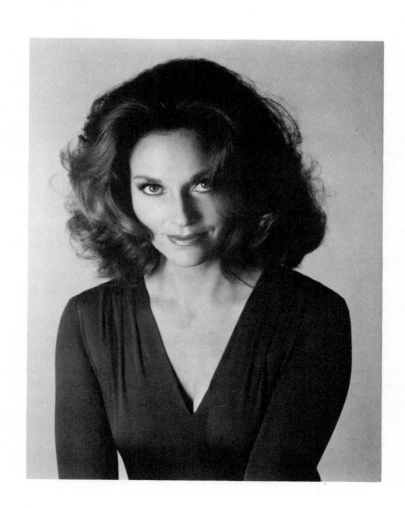

# A Word from Lee Meriwether

Practically everyone is now aware of the value of good nutrition and regular exercise. If there are any secrets to radiant health and beauty, they must certainly be found in self-help procedures that improve health. This timely and fascinating book drawn from the combined talents of Peter Lupus and Dr. Samuel Homola reveals these secrets freely and openly.

With the trend back to natural foods and natural methods gaining momentum every day, this book will give you a head start in using natural beauty-building procedures that will soon be universally acclaimed.

My work in front of cameras and on the stage has made me acutely aware of the need for a simple but effective health-and-beauty program that yields *permanent* results. Happily, this useful book by Mr. Lupus and Dr. Homola offers such a program. I recommend it for every woman who wants to feel better and look better.

*Lee Meriwether*

# A Foreword–
# Frank S. Caprio, M.D.

This book, undoubtedly by virtue of the title alone, is destined to have a well-deserved wide readership, especially among women who have a sincere and genuine desire to improve themselves in every way. It can now be accomplished via an easy-to-follow total health program. The authors cover an extensive range of topics, all related to the central theme of "radiant health and beauty," and they include a separate chapter devoted to ways the average woman can experience the sexual fulfillment that is so essential to overall physical and emotional health.

It is a medically sound, inspirational do-it-yourself book written in simple, nontechnical language, and it furnishes practical, common-sense guidance as to how women everywhere can stay young, keep well, and enjoy life—how they can achieve better living through better thinking. I am in complete accord with the authors when they contend that to *feel* well you must *think* well. This implies safeguarding your health and general well-being.

Each chapter represents a valuable lesson in self-improvement and successful living.

Peter Lupus and Dr. Samuel Homola are to be congratulated for offering so many women an opportunity to acquire the knowledge they need for the development of a better way of life—*healthier, happier, and sex-cessful.*

Becoming increasingly attractive and beautiful *inwardly* as well as *outwardly* is but a way of living. It's all a matter of *mental attitude* and what

10

you intend to do about yourself as a result of reading this book. It's as simple as that.

Every woman needs to convince herself of her right to happiness, her right to be good to herself, to make life *easier* and more self-satisfying and enjoyable, to make day-to-day self-improvement as outlined in this book a *lifetime resolution.*

The unique and medically sound programs offered by Mr. Lupus and Dr. Homola have been presented in what is undoubtedly the most useful and complete health-and-beauty book ever written exclusively for women. It will make a valuable addition to your library, and it will change your life for the better.

*Frank S. Caprio M.D.*

# What This Book Is And What It Is Not

Would you like to improve your health and your physical appearance? Do you wish you were more beautiful and more desirable? If your answer to any part of either of these questions is "yes," you need this book.

No matter how physically deprived you may feel you are, you can improve your physical appearance with such simple measures as diet and exercise. You can, in fact, expect a *miraculous* transformation in your physical appearance if you follow the programs outlined in this book. Best of all, you'll improve your health, and, with an improvement in health, you'll automatically become more beautiful.

Remember that you cannot be truly beautiful if you are not healthy. Use of cosmetics and other artificial beautification methods cannot conceal unhealthy skin, brittle hair, excess fat, flabby muscles, and other signs of poor health. For this reason, this book is not concerned with beauty shop procedures. There are many available beauty books that offer instructions in the use of cosmetics and other temporary beauty aids. It's perfectly all right to use such aids. Every woman does. A little carefully applied make-up can be very appealing. But you should first learn how to improve your health and your physical appearance with methods that will make you *permanently* beautiful.

## A Complete Guide for Women

In this book you'll learn how to *change* your physical appearance with simple health-building procedures. Chapters on nutrition, exercise, body development, skin care, and self-improvement provide a complete handbook for every woman who wants to be healthy, beautiful, and desirable. Special material on cellulite, reducing, sex, and other subjects of special interest to women makes this one of the most helpful books ever written exclusively for women. Read it carefully. Put into practice what you learn and you'll be surprised and pleased with the results. You'll be healthier and happier.

With this book you can get the guidance *you* need to be physically beautiful. And, with an improvement in health, you'll *feel* beautiful.

*Samuel Homola*

*Peter Lupus*

# Contents

# any woman can become more beautiful and more desirable!

There isn't anything more beautiful than a beautiful woman! At least that's the opinion of the authors of this book. The most beautiful woman, however, is not necessarily the most desirable. So it's often not enough just to be beautiful. You can be both beautiful *and* desirable if you follow the programs outlined in this book.

## Beauty Is a Whole Person

You want to be your most attractive and desirable self, whether to advance your career, please the men in your life, or just to feel good about yourself. In the eyes of many men, a beautiful woman is automatically desirable. This is, of course, a judgment made on a purely physical basis. We all know that a beautiful woman is not always the best wife or mate. Once the physical fires have cooled and the novelty has worn off, there must be something else to hold a man and a woman together in a permanent relationship. This "something else" is not as obvious as physical beauty, but it's important. A beautiful woman who is constantly sick, for example, or who is "frigid" because of an improper attitude toward sex, may find it difficult to hold the attention of the average man for very long. Beauty cannot be substituted for passion, compassion, personality, and other qualities. So an improvement in health and attitude can be just as important as cultivating a shapely calf in winning and holding a worthwhile man.

16

# Chapter 1

## A Program Designed Especially for Women

Since this book has been written especially for women, it will deal solely with programs that are designed to make every woman more beautiful and more desirable. This means that the subject matter of this book will cover a great variety of material, from nutrition to sex. You"ll learn how to use natural foods, vitamin E, special diets, and other popular health measures that you've heard about.

If you follow *all* the programs outlined in this book, you'll benefit in many ways other than attracting the attention of men. In addition to becoming more beautiful, for example, you'll have healthier children and you'll live longer. Aging will be slowed, so that you won't look as old as other women your age.

## Follow the Example of Shari Lewis

When you neglect your body, you're hurting yourself in many ways. Shari Lewis, the lovely and multi-talented star of "The Shari Show," fully realizes the importance of taking good care of her body. "I started as a dancer," she recalls, "And early in my teens, I realized that I was my own instrument—which meant that anything I did to hurt myself would ruin the only thing I had to offer—*me*."

Every star realizes that it's "good business" to stay healthy. It's just as important for *you* to stay healthy if you want to enjoy life and live fully. After all, all you really have is *you*—and what you have to offer is *you*. So be kind to yourself and pamper your body.

## Every Woman Is Unique and Special

Remember that no matter how beautiful you are or may become, you'll have to use good judgment in selecting a man who does not judge you on physical beauty alone. You have much more to offer than your body. You have something *special* that no other woman has. Every woman is unique in her own way. The type of man who fails to see each woman as an individual, and who is attracted only by physical beauty, does not make the best husband or mate.

Even if you have the ideal man, you owe it to yourself and to him to do all you can to improve your health and your physical appearance. A poorly cared-for body reflects a form of negligence that can be expected to extend into all phases of life. Besides, bad health resulting from physical negligence can result in much pain, suffering, and expense. Physical deterioration of your body can be embarrassing to you and repulsive to those around you. You'll get along better in this world, and you'll score better in the mating game, if you'll take good care of your body.

### Improving Your Physical Appearance Can Change Your Life! It Did for Annette!

The experience of Annette B. is a good example of how an improvement in physical appearance can change someone's life. Annette was 24 years of age, jobless, unmarried, and overweight. She was obviously unhealthy, and she had a defensive, pessimistic attitude that alienated everyone who knew her. Since she was resigned to a boring, lonely life, she didn't care how she looked. "I am what I am," she insisted, "and there isn't anything I can do about it."

A neighbor loaned Annette a copy of a popular health book, much like the one you're now reading. For the first time, Annette realized that she might be able to do something about her physical appearance. She got on a "health kick" and started eating natural foods. Miraculously, she began to lose weight. As if by magic, the color of her skin improved. Her hair quit breaking off at the roots and grew stronger and thicker. Annette felt so much better that she started swimming and playing tennis. The changes that took place in her physical appearance were almost unbelievable. In six months, she changed from a pale, tired, cranky, overweight "old woman" to a slim, tanned, vivacious, and beautiful girl.

"My own parents didn't recognize me when I visited them this summer!" she exclaimed. "My new way of life has literally made a different person of me."

Annette *was* a different person. She looked different and felt different. Even her attitude changed. And, as she became more popular and more confident, she became more ambitious. She got a job in a bank, joined a tennis club, and married an Air Force pilot.

Annette's story sounds like a Cinderella tale, but it's true, and she owes it all to her efforts to improve her health and her physical appearance.

### Lee Meriwether: The Ultimate Success Story

Every woman dreams of winning the No. 1 beauty contest and then stepping into stardom in movies and television. Few women can ever hope to accomplish such a feat, and most place such dreams in the realm of fantasy. But Lee Meriwether, a former "Miss America" now co-starring in the "Barnaby Jones" television series, made these dreams come true. And in a great variety of roles in movies and on the stage, she has displayed a rare combination of beauty and talent that has won the admiration of men and women alike.

Like most successful women, Lee Meriwether does not take her success for granted. In addition to continued effort in developing her acting and singing talents, she pays close attention to her personal health program. She eats *natural* foods, with emphasis on fresh fruits and vegetables. And to make sure that she gets adequate amounts of the nutrients she needs to preserve her beauty and to combat aging, she supplements her diet with vitamins A, C, and E.

How does she stay so physically trim? When she isn't spending 12 to 14 hours a day filming a movie, she gets her exercise by attending two-hour dance classes three or four times a week. She also plays tennis, and whenever possible she jogs for 15 minutes four or five times a week.

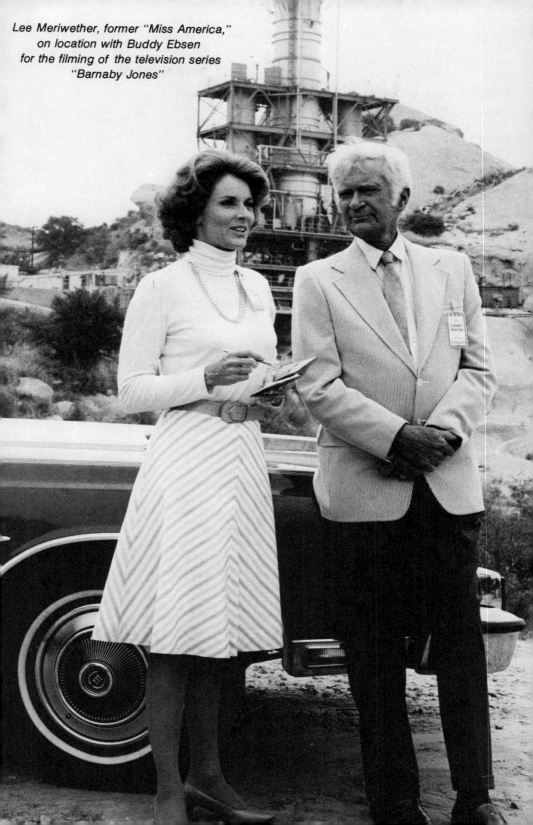

Lee Meriwether, former "Miss America,"
on location with Buddy Ebsen
for the filming of the television series
"Barnaby Jones"

Lee Meriwether stays beautiful and healthy by eating properly, taking supplements, and exercising regularly, just as you'll be advised to do in this book. She emphasizes, however, that the power of positive thinking can have much to do with what you are and what you become. "Any woman can become more beautiful," she advises, "if she will say to herself 'I'm beautiful in my own way' and really believe it."

So even if you don't win a beauty contest or become a movie star, you can be beautiful and successful in your own special way. Remember, however, that it's absolutely essential that you take the best possible care of your health and your body—and that's what this book is all about.

### How a Diet-and-Exercise Program Can Improve Your Health and Your Physical Appearance

There is no better way to make fast, dramatic changes in your physical appearance than to embark on a carefully planned diet and exercise program. The proper diet can remove *all* the excess fat from your body. Special exercises can actually *change* your body shape by toning and molding skeletal muscles. There are many diet and exercise programs on the market. Some are effective and some aren't. Some are actually dangerous. You won't find any harmful fads in this book. Instead, you'll receive instructions in *safe* diet and exercise methods that have been proven to be effective for stars, celebrities, and other persons who need the best possible results in the fastest possible time.

Remember that exercise is only a small part of the total program offered in this book. If you don't feel that you need to exercise, you may simply study the material on the nutrition, body care, sex technique, and other subjects in which you have special interest.

You'll learn in chapter 2 how to reduce your bodyweight with a generous diet of delicious natural foods. This same diet will improve your health and prolong your life. If you've been reading the newspapers lately, you know that the fiber supplied by natural foods may help to prevent such diseases as colon cancer, diverticulitis, and appendicitis. You can be a part of the trend back to natural foods by using natural foods to reduce your bodyweight. And just to make sure that you get maximum nutrients with minimum calories, chapter 3 will tell you how to *prepare* natural foods.

Even if you aren't overweight, you should limit your diet to natural foods. Simply eliminating refined and processed foods from your diet will often prevent a gain in bodyweight. But you must have a balanced diet made up of the basic natural foods for good health.

### Keeping Yourself Young

As you grow older, your health will become more important to you than beauty. If you want to stay healthy and live a long time, you'll have to begin taking care of your health *now*, and you'll have to adopt a program that you can follow for a lifetime. *If you stay healthy, you'll stay beautiful.*

Chapter 12 will tell you exactly what you must do to keep yourself youthful. What you learn in chapters 2 and 3 about selecting and preparing natural foods is also an important part of your longevity program. So be sure to study *all* of the material in this book.

### A Good Sex Life Builds Good Health

There are many bonuses in good health. Your sex life, for example, will improve when your health improves. You'll be more vivacious as well as more appealing and more passionate. Sex itself is a wholesome, healthful activity. A satisfying sex life can, by itself, improve your health.

You'll learn more about how to have a happy, successful sex life when you read chapter 10. And what you learn might surprise you. Did you know, for example, that there are many women who have never had a sexual climax? Every woman can and should have a regular orgasm. But each woman has to *make* it happen. If you believe that the climax of lovemaking is a "spiritual thing that happens only with the right man," you have been misinformed. No matter how much you love your man or how good a lover he might be, your ability to have an orgasm is primarily up to you. You have to make a deliberate effort to reach the ecstasy of a sexual climax.

Spiritual love helps, and love makes sex more beautiful. But *technique* is the key to sexual orgasm. So brace yourself for instructions in basic sexual techniques. With new knowledge and a change in attitude, you can experience a whole new world of pleasure.

If your love life is not what is should be, with or without a man, you'll appreciate chapter 10. In the meantime, remember that you can satisfy a man best by concentrating on satisfying yourself.

### Every Woman Can Benefit from Food Supplements

Surveys indicate that the average person is deficient in one or more of the essential nutrients. One reason for this, of course, is that fresh, natural foods are not readily available to everyone. Processing and improper preparation of foods result in the loss of many essential nutrients.

Stress, air pollution, and other factors destroy nutrients in the body, creating deficiencies even when the diet is basically good. Did you know, for example, that when you are under stress you need larger amounts of vitamin C? Or that air pollution raises your requirement for vitamin E?

You should try to get all the essential nutrients from the foods you eat. Unless you live on an isolated farm in a carefully controlled environment, however, it's not likely that you'll get adequate amounts of certain nutrients. For this reason, it might be a good idea to take certain basic vitamin and mineral supplements, with emphasis on nutrients known to be commonly deficient in women. Young women who menstruate heavily, for example, might need to take an iron supplement. Women who take birth control pills are often deficient in vitamin B6. Menopausal women often need extra calcium to prevent the development of a "dowager's hump" and other symptoms of soft bones.

You'll learn in chapter 4 how to use vitamins and minerals in building and restoring good health. In chapter 5, you'll get all the information you need on how to use special natural food supplements for quick and inexpensive sources of certain essential nutrients. When you finish reading these two chapters, you'll be an authority on food supplements for women.

### Lucille Ball: A Skiing Accident Changed Her Life

If you could see superstar Lucille Ball do high kicks, you'd never believe that this vivacious woman once suffered a serious leg fracture that was complicated by a nutritional deficiency. How could that happen? Let Lucy explain.

"In January of 1972," she related in a personal interview, "I was just standing on a ski slope with the instructor and a few other people. I was putting on my gloves when a woman standing next to me began to fall. She grabbed my pole to hold herself up and took me with her when she fell. She just landed on her fanny, but I was screwed into the ground."

This simple stress on Lucy's legs fractured the bones in her right thigh and lower leg! X-ray examination revealed that she was suffering from osteoporosis, a calcium deficiency that results in soft, brittle bones.

"I had never exercised regularly," Lucy admitted, "and I never took vitamins and minerals and didn't think about my nutrition until my skiing accident."

Today, Lucille Ball takes 24 vitamin and mineral capsules each morning to supplement "simple, well-balanced meals,"

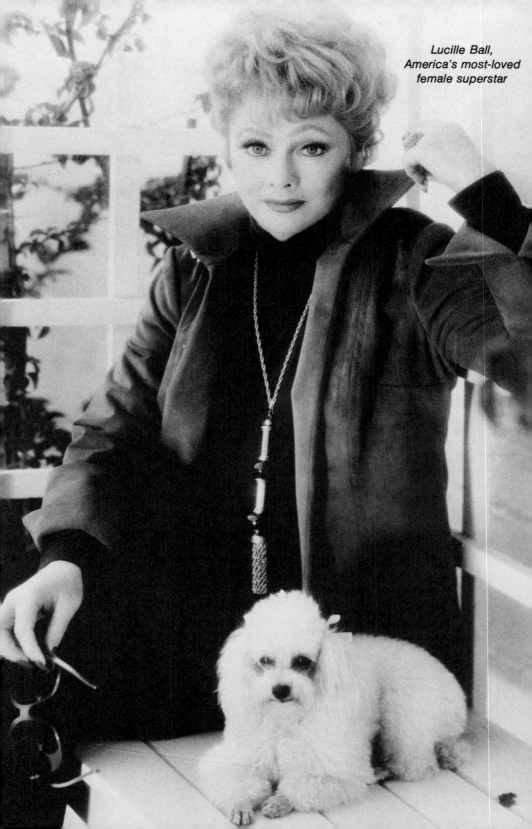

*Lucille Ball, America's most-loved female superstar*

and she rarely fails to take some form of exercise each day. "Too many people are overwhelmed by the thought of exercising," she observed, "and they don't like to go to a gym. But, believe me, you can do most exercises at home, even if you can't build a workout area in your house. . . . I can't ski anymore, but I can *walk* cross country on skis. Now when I don't work out every day I miss it."

Lucy presently weighs 135 pounds and is stronger and healthier than ever. And that's good news! We all love Lucy and hope to see more of her in the future.

You can benefit from Lucille Ball's experience and *prevent* the development of osteoporosis by carrying out the recommendations outlined in this book. Chapter 13 describes many simple exercises that you can do at home.

### Special Care for Skin and Hair Problems

Regardless of how healthy you might be, you may have to use special procedures in caring for your skin, hair, and nails. Take skin, for example. No two people have skin that is exactly alike. Skin can be oily, dry, or "normal." There are various degrees of oily and dry skin. Each type must be cared for differently. Bad skin can add years to your physical appearance.

With proper skin care, you can preserve the youthfulness of your skin so that you won't become dry and wrinkled as you mature. Actually, skin care is very simple. You don't need a great variety of expensive cosmetics. You can care for almost any type of skin with proper use of soap, water, vegetable oil, and lemon juice.

You'll learn in chapter 6 how to care for your skin, hair, and nails so that their natural beauty will be preserved for a lifetime.

### Teeth Should Last Forever

Loss of teeth is one of the most horrible things that can happen to any woman. Yet, almost every woman past middle age suffers from loss of teeth. Many women begin to lose their teeth before they reach 40 years of age. Half of all persons over the age of 55 do not have any natural teeth!

There's a simple explanation for premature loss of teeth. And there's *plenty* that you can do to *prevent* such a loss. In fact, there's no reason why you cannot keep your teeth as long as you live.

What you learn in chapter 7 about caring for your teeth will be price-less in preserving the beauty of your mouth.

### A New Solution to the Old Problem of Lumpy Fat

Just about every woman develops lumpy fat around her hips and thighs. This unattractive fat, called "cellulite," is so common that it re-ceives special attention in expensive spas where reducing is a specialty. Since it is believed that cellulite is not ordinary fat, however, something more than a reducing diet is usually recommended as a "cure."

Chapter 8 will tell you how to get rid of lumpy fat by using procedures that will improve your health as well as beautify your body.

### Special Solutions for Special Problems

Do you have a bony chest, small breasts, sagging buttocks, or some other body problem? You may be able to find a solution for your problem in chapter 8. You can use special exercises, for example, to fill in bony areas and lift up sagging body parts. A simple change in posture is often all that's needed to lift up a pot belly or to take the slump out of your back. All this information has been placed in the same chapter that tells you how to get rid of cellulite, so that you can put it all together to make wonderful changes in your body.

### Build a New Body with Weight Training

If you're slim and bony or flabby and saggy and you feel that you'd like to trade your old body for a new one, try a little weight training. *There's no better way to mold a new figure than to exercise with barbells and dumbbells.* Even if you feel that you already have a good figure, you can keep it that way with only a small amount of resistance exercise or weight training. Remember that it's your *muscles* that shape your soft, feminine curves. Without the support of well-developed muscles, your body fat would sag grotesquely.

You don't need to worry about getting too muscular from weight training. Your female hormones will prevent excessive muscular de-velopment. Every woman can follow the weight-training program outlined in chapter 9, with predictably good results.

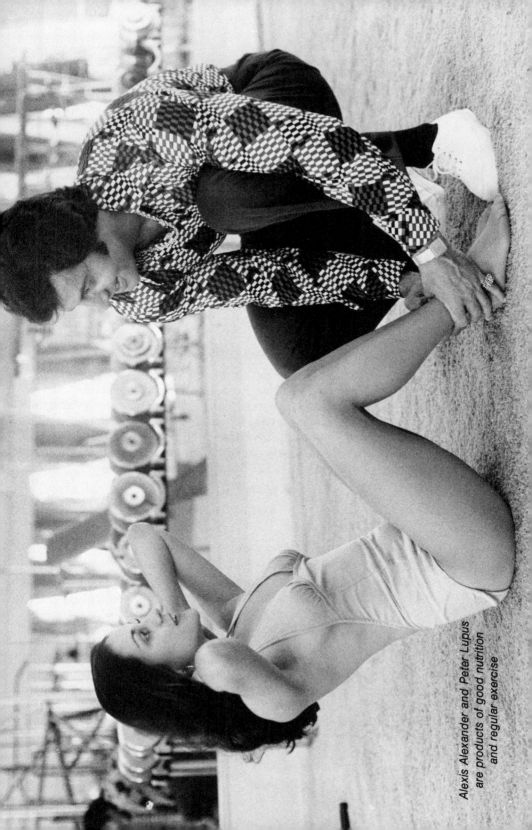

Alexis Alexander and Peter Lupus are products of good nutrition and regular exercise

### Spring Back from Pregnancy or Illness

We've all seen beautiful, young women who seem to deteriorate physically after illness or after giving birth to a child. You cannot always avoid illness. If you follow a good health program, however, you can prevent many forms of illness. You can certainly increase your resistance against disease and infection, and with a healthy body you'll recover more rapidly from illness. A special program, like the one recommended in chapter 11, will help you regain your youthful appearance following illness or pregnancy. The same program will *prepare* you for pregnancy.

Every woman who wants children should be able to have them without fear of losing her beauty or her health. Without good health and a strong body, however, both the mother and the child are endangered during pregnancy.

### You Can Prevent the Development of Disease

The average woman outlives her man, but women, like men, usually die from disease rather than from old age. *Almost all the leading dangerous diseases could be prevented with proper attention to good health habits*. Heart disease and cancer, for example, are often considered the result of bad eating habits. The same program you use to build your health and improve your physical appearance will help prevent many common illnesses. Chapter 12 will tell you how to slow the aging process, but what you learn in *every chapter* of this book will help prevent the development of disease.

### You Can Be Healthy and Still Have a Good Time!

Following a good health program doesn't mean that you have to be some kind of fanatic. You can, in fact, have as much fun as anyone else. After you have finished reading this book, you'll know how to be selective in what you eat and drink when you go out on the town. And if you're sensible enough to be moderate in an occasional spree, you can join a party without hurting your health. But you have to be *original*. You have to be a little different from everyone else. Remember that if you want to stay youthful, beautiful, desirable, and live a long time, you can't live like all the people you know who are suffering from poor health, aging prematurely, and dying from disease.

The rewards of good living habits are well worth the few small sacrifices you have to make. So don't feel too sorry for yourself because you

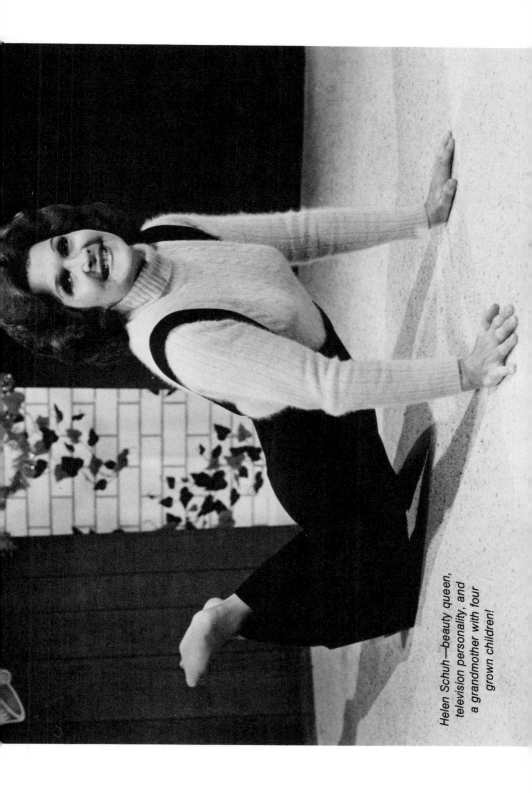

Helen Schuh—beauty queen, television personality, and a grandmother with four grown children!

can't allow yourself to keep up with the bad habits of some of your friends. Natural foods, sex, and all the other good things of life can give you more pleasure than a steady diet of bad habits.

### Special Exercises to Improve Your Sex Life

For the first time in any book, chapter 13 describes some original, nationally televised exercises that you can do at home to improve your sex life as well as your physical appearance! You'll have fun doing these exercises, and you'll want to show your partner and your friends how to do them.

### How to Win a Man with Actions and Attitude

No matter how youthful or beautiful you might be, you won't be fully appreciated if you do not have a good personal relationship with your man. A woman who does not respect her man or encourage him, for example, might not be able to beat the competition of a homely woman who inflates a man's ego.

Sexual response is also important. A plain woman who enjoys sex is going to be much more attractive than a cold beauty who is irritated by sexual activity. A woman who truly loves her man will get a great deal of satisfaction from pleasing him sexually, even if she does not herself reach a sexual climax.

Of course, one of the first requirements for a good relationship with a man is to find a man who is not too chauvinistic or self-centered to appreciate the qualities of a good woman. If you find the right man, you can love him, please him, respect him and be devoted to him, and get equal treatment in return.

You'll learn more about how to be appreciated at home when you read chapter 14. In the meantime, remember that if your man feels that you really admire him and desire him, he'll feel that you are the most desirable woman in the world. As Jackie Gleason says, a desirable woman is one who tells her man, "You're the greatest!"

Your *mental attitude* has much to do with your happiness and your relationship with people. If you're a victim of stress and tension, and it's affecting your state of mind, you'll appreciate the tips in chapter 14 on how to control stress and overcome nervous tension.

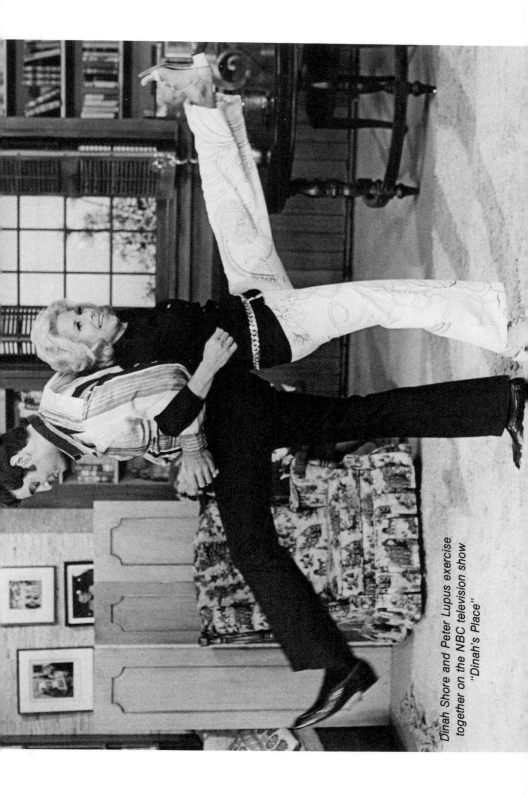

Dinah Shore and Peter Lupus exercise together on the NBC television show "Dinah's Place"

### Dinah Shore—a Truly Desirable Woman

Ask any man to name a woman who best exemplifies a desirable southern female and chances are he'll say, "Dinah Shore." This beautiful, friendly, and relaxed woman has a way of making the men around her feel masculine and important. Dinah readily admits that she thinks of her life as incomplete unless she is sharing it with a man she loves. Even if she were not famous and beautiful, her attitude and her manner would still make her attractive and desirable to men. (The Gallup Poll has repeatedly listed Dinah Shore among the "Ten Most Admired Women in the World.")

Miss Shore stays physically beautiful by staying physically fit. Since she does not enjoy exercising for the sake of exercising, she prefers such recreational exercise as golf and tennis. Many of the exercises described in chapter 13 of this book have been demonstrated in partner-fun fashion by Dinah Shore and Peter Lupus on the NBC television show "Dinah's Place."

"Stay active," Dinah advises, "if you want beauty eternal, and never overeat." If you've read Dinah Shore's cookbook, *Someone's in the Kitchen with Dinah,* you know that she is a gourmet cook. But she obviously doesn't overeat, and she uses exercise for added protection against a buildup of body fat.

It's not Dinah's cooking, however, that makes her so appealing to men; it's her *attitude.* Take a lesson from Dinah and cultivate a warm, friendly attitude to enhance your physical beauty.

## Plan Ahead for Your Later Years

Following the instructions in this book will prepare you physically for a long and healthy life. But when you reach retirement age, you must stay mentally and physically active with hobbies and other activities that will give your life pleasure and purpose. The final chapter of this book will give you a few tips on how to begin preparing for your mature years *now.*

### Step into a New Way of Life as Louisa Recommends

Beautiful Louisa Biedenharn, owner and operator of the fabulous Louisa Health and Beauty Resort, has observed

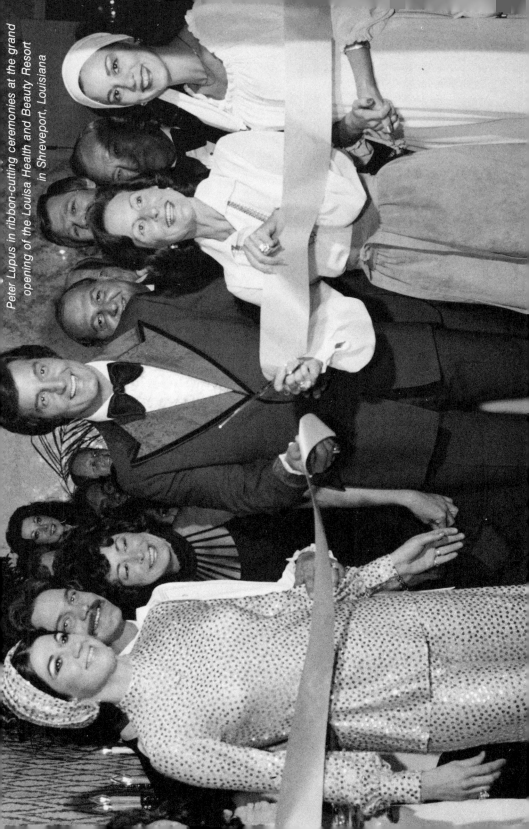

Peter Lupus in ribbon-cutting ceremonies at the grand opening of the Louisa Health and Beauty Resort in Shreveport, Louisiana that there is a close connection between mental and physical health. During almost two decades of working in the health-and-beauty field, she has personally witnessed the miraculous transformation that takes place in the minds and bodies of women who undertake a program to improve their health and their physical appearance. Her popular resort in Shreveport, Louisiana, is considered by many to be the finest and most luxurious health-and-beauty resort ever opened exclusively for women.

Utilizing programs endorsed by Peter Lupus, Louisa recommends good nutrition along with regular exercise in a complete program. "At my resort," she emphasizes, "we stress a sensible diet and use a well-rounded program of regular exercise to aid weight control, help overcome chronic fatigue, improve the functioning of the heart and lungs, prolong the active years, and virtually make life interesting and full of excitement at any age. The results have been startling! Changed personalities sparkle with healthy good looks. Improved figures, young and limber, move with ease and grace. A fascinating inner glow reflects health and vigor that make each woman more interesting and exciting.

"Every woman should start *today* to develop a life-long program to keep herself more feminine, naturally beautiful, lovelier to look at, and, most of all, desirable and exciting to be with, regardless of age."

You can "cut the ribbon" and step into a new way of life by turning the page and reading chapter 2 of this book, which has been written especially for *you.*

## SUMMARY

1. With the right program, *every woman* can become more beautiful and more desirable.

2. The first chapter of this book is only a preview of what you'll find in other chapters of this book.

3. If you follow the *complete* program outlined in this book, you'll improve your health and lengthen your life as well as become more beautiful.

4. Every chapter of this book has many surprises, and the good health that results from what you learn reading this book will benefit you for the rest of your life.

5. Take the second step in your beautification program and begin reading chapter 2.

# some celebrity diets and how they work

Overweight is a common complaint among today's women. (It's a problem for men, too! But remember that this book has been written strictly for women.) Most women are concerned only about the effect of overweight on their physical appearance. An overweight body can be just as damaging to health as to physical beauty, however. Did you know, for example, that diabetes, arthritis, heart disease, hardened arteries, high blood pressure, cancer, kidney ailments, varicose veins, hernia, gall bladder trouble, and other common ailments have often been related to obesity? If you reduce or control your bodyweight with a balanced diet of fresh, natural foods, you'll be able to *prevent* the development of many diseases. You'll also eliminate some of the leading causes of death.

So even if you aren't overweight, you should follow the dietary recommendations outlined in this chapter in order to protect your health as well as to stay slim and trim.

Remember this ancient Egyptian proverb: "We live off a quarter of all we eat. Doctors live off the other three quarters." An anonymous wit has since summed up the situation: "Eat less, but eat well, so you can live longer to eat more."

## Every Woman Should Avoid Sugar and Refined Carbohydrates

Many overweight people habitually eat excessive amounts of sugar and white-flour products. The average person eats more than 115 pounds

# Chapter 2

of sugar each year! The average diet is *loaded* with refined carbohydrates that supply empty calories. It's no wonder that so many people are overweight! *Simply eliminating sugar and white-flour products from the diet would, in most cases, result in a loss of weight.* Conversely, inclusion of only a small amount of sugar or refined carbohydrate in a reducing diet may make it difficult or impossible to lose weight. And here's why: When sugar or refined carbohydrate is eaten, a sudden rise in blood sugar places a load on the pancreas. Normally, the pancreas secretes just enough insulin to remove the excess blood sugar for storage. When the pancreas has been overworked by an overload day after day, however, it may develop a sensitivity that causes it to overreact to any sudden rise in blood sugar. The result is that so much sugar is removed from the blood that the body is forced to store blood sugar as fat, leaving very little to be burned for energy. This is why some fat people are always hungry and tired, even though they are constantly snacking on sweets and refined carbohydrates.

### Jeanette's Bout with Overweight

At the age of 33, Jeanette C. was an overweight housewife who had been overweight since her graduation from high school. After 13 years of marriage, she was heavier than ever.

"I try to count my calories," she maintained, "but it doesn't seem to do any good. I've gained two pounds this month! But I don't see how. I'm so starved that I often feel weak and shaky. I get so hungry between meals that I just have to have a sandwich, but when I do eat between meals I eat less at mealtime."

A look at Jeanette's diet revealed that she did, indeed, eat very little, but what she did eat was largely processed and refined. For example, she often had refined cereal and white bread toast for breakfast, potato chips and hamburgers for lunch, and commercial pot pies with coffee in the evening. When Jeanette limited her diet to the type of foods recommended in this chapter, she started to lose weight even though she ate more. And just to make sure that her blood sugar did not fluctuate, she had between-meal snacks of fresh fruit and cottage cheese. "I've been losing weight steadily now for the last three months," she reported. "And I haven't had any more spells with my nerves. Best of all, I have more energy than I've ever had, and I'm more alert. I now actually look forward to getting up each morning!"

Jeanette was able to take in more calories and lose weight primarily because she eliminated refined carbohydrates from her diet. The change in her energy level was, of course, the result of normalization of her blood sugar. As a result of shedding pounds of ugly fat, Jeanette's personality changed along with her body. She developed an aggressive new interest in the pleasures of living—and people developed a new interest in *her*.

If you're really serious about reducing your bodyweight and getting a new lease on life, you, too, should try to avoid using sugar and white-flour products. Even if you don't suffer from a pancreatic sensitivity, you can reduce your weight *faster* if you exclude the empty calories supplied by refined carbohydrates.

### Coffee Breaks and Low Blood Sugar

Many people who suffer from hypoglycemia (low blood sugar) must have high-protein snacks *between meals* to keep their blood sugar up and to avoid a craving for sweets. It may also be necessary to avoid drinking coffee, tea, and cola. The caffeine in these beverages can cause a sudden rise in blood sugar by stimulating the adrenal glands. The pancreas may then overreact, just as it does when sugar is eaten, forcing the body to store blood sugar as fat.

Stick to beverages that do not require sweetening. Drink fruit and vegetable juices, skimmed milk, and water. Drink *water* when you are thirsty. Remember that when you are on a reducing diet you need plenty of water to help your kidneys flush out waste products.

Try to avoid using artificial sweeteners. Since the body cannot metabolize or eliminate the chemicals in such sweeteners, they tend to accumulate in the liver and other organs where they may have harmful effects.

### Stay Active and Avoid Counting Calories

If you limit your diet to properly prepared natural foods, it's not likely that you'll overeat. Natural foods won't artificially stimulate your appetite. And chances are your appetite mechanism will let you know when you have had enough to eat. If you exercise regularly, it would actually be difficult to take in too many calories on a diet of natural foods. All you have to do is stop eating when you are comfortably satisfied.

### Eat to Satisfy Your Appetite

Dorina T. was so pudgy that she was too embarrassed to attend a swimming class with her children. She wanted to lose weight, but since her husband was a construction worker who had a big appetite, she was reluctant to go on a low-calorie diet. "I have to cook for my husband and I want to eat with him," she insisted, "so I want to eat the same foods if possible."

Chances are Dorina could have fed her husband and trimmed her weight down simply by following the eight basic rules outlined later in this chapter. But just to make sure that she could eat generously without counting calories, she followed the basic rules and played tennis twice a week. She lost 20 pounds in two months, in spite of eating to satisfy her appetite! Her body firmed up beautifully, allowing her to wear revealing new dresses and swimsuits. An improvement in her health actually thickened her hair and increased her pep and vitality. "My only problem now," she complained tongue-in-cheek, "is that my husband won't leave me alone. He's so turned on by my new physical appearance that he feels as if he's having an affair with another woman!"

Whenever possible, do as Dorina did and participate in some form of recreational exercise when you go on a diet. You're bound to lose weight if you exercise regularly and eat properly. You'll certainly *look* better than someone who loses weight with diet alone.

### Advice from Shirley MacLaine

Award-winning actress Shirley MacLaine lost 30 pounds in six months simply by "returning to proper foods at regular meals" and by getting plenty of exercise in yoga and ballet. She offers this advice for women starting a reducing program: "Give yourself a sense of hope. . . . Be consistent in actions you've promised yourself to take, and be patient about results."

Now 42 years of age, Shirley MacLaine is still slim, trim, and beautiful, and she is as energetic and flexible as a teenager. She also has a brilliant mind, and is the author of the best-selling book *Don't Fall Off the Mountain.*

## How to Reduce Your Bodyweight with Food Fiber

In addition to being rich in beauty-building nutrients, natural foods are rich in fiber that will help you reduce you bodyweight. The fiber in whole-grain products, for example, will actually interfere with absorption of calories. A slice of whole-grain bread contains about the same number of calories as a slice of white bread, but you'll absorb fewer calories from the whole-grain bread. Fiber in fresh fruits and vegetables, in the form of cellulose, allows you to eat greater quantities of these foods without gaining weight.

Even if you are not overweight, there are a couple of good reasons why you should not eat processed foods if you can avoid them. There is now some evidence to indicate that too much refined sugar in the diet can contribute to the development of bowel cancer by altering the bacterial content of the lower colon. And when there is not enough fiber or roughage in the diet, delayed emptying of the bowels can allow bacterial activity to convert bile acids into cancer-causing chemicals.

If you eat plenty of fresh fruits and vegetables and whole-grain products, your bowels will empty before harmful chemicals can form. It'll be easier to reduce your bodyweight.

### How Rose Marie Improved Her Health with Fiber

Rose Marie B., a 48-year-old department store clerk, weighed 158 pounds when she began to suffer from recurring cramps in the lower left-hand side of her abdomen. When she wasn't constipated she suffered from diarrhea. An x-ray examination revealed that she had diverticulitis, or inflammation of numerous small pouches in the walls of her colon. Her doctor put her on a soft, or low-residue, diet consisting of such foods as milk, refined cereals, eggs, white bread, and potatoes, which contain practically no fiber. The result was that she *gained weight,* and she continued to suffer from constipation, diarrhea, and abdominal pain.

When Rose Marie switched to a diet of natural foods, as recommended in this chapter, her bowel problems disappeared almost immediately. Over a period of six months, she reduced her weight from 186 pounds to 146 pounds! "Thank goodness I got rid of that large, rumbling stomach," she said gratefully, patting her flat abdomen. "It was bad enough to be fat, but it was worse to have my day spoiled by constipation or diarrhea."

Doctors now know that bran or fiber in the diet sweeps the bowel clean and prevents formation or clogging of diverticula or colon pouches. The type of diet that supplies adequate fiber usually also supplies the nutrients you need to improve your health while you reduce your bodyweight.

### *How to Increase Your Intake of Fiber*

You can add additional fiber to your diet by sprinkling bran over cereals and other foods or by mixing it into homemade bread (see chapter 3) or meat loaf. You can purchase pure, unprocessed bran in any health food store. Use at least a couple of tablespoons daily, but don't overdo it. Since bran does not supply nutrients, it should not be used as a substitute for food. Remember that your bowels need the cellulose supplied by raw fruits and vegetables just as much as they need the fiber supplied by bran. About two teaspoons of bran with each meal should be about right for most people.

Begin your bran program by taking two teaspoons of bran with your evening meal. If no adverse effects occur, such as loose bowels, work your way up to six teaspoons daily (two with each meal). Use as much bran as necessary to maintain good bowel function. (Although bran is indigestible, it is "softage" rather than roughage and will not normally irritate the bowel. It simply provides moisture-holding bulk that is made up of *soft* fiber. So don't be afraid to use it.) Drink plenty of water so that the fiber in your bowels will stay moist. A couple of glasses of water between meals would be helpful. Adding bran and water to your diet will help curb your appetite by filling your stomach with zero-calorie bulk.

Try to eat a little yogurt each day. The lactobacillus (bacteria) supplied by yogurt will help curtail the activity of the harmful bacteria in your colon. (If you have a blood sugar problem that compels you to have a high-protein snack between meals, yogurt will fill the bill.)

### The Seven Basic Food Groups

No matter what type of diet you go on, you should make sure that you eat some of *all* the basic foods in order to get the nutrients your body needs to be healthy and beautiful. If you can't eat something from each of the seven basic food groups every day, try to include them all over a period of two days. For example, you can eat fruits one day and vegetables the next day. Or you can alternate the meat group with the skimmed milk group, and so on.

Every natural food contains a variety of essential nutrients. No one food item is indispensable. But you must make sure that you get the nutrients you need from the various food groups. For example, you must eat animal or dairy products for the vitamin $B_{12}$ you need to prevent anemia. You need the iodine supplied by ocean fish or seafood. It's difficult to get enough calcium without using milk products. And, of course, you *must* have the fiber supplied by whole-grain products if you want to prevent diseases of the intestinal tract. You'll automatically get the nutrients you need if you'll simply base your diet on the seven basic food groups.

You'll learn in chapter 3 how to prepare foods for maximum nutrients with minimum calories. In the meantime, just remember not to use grease or oil in preparing any of the foods in these groups.

Here are the seven basic food groups:

**1. Green and yellow vegetables** (for vitamin A and cellulose). You may eat generous amounts of any vegetable in this group.

**2. Citrus fruit, tomatoes, and raw cabbage** (for vitamin C and cellulose). The foods in this group should always be eaten raw. You can include many of your favorite vegetables in a raw salad.

**3. Potatoes and other vegetables and fruits** (for natural carbohydrate). Even though you must eliminate refined carbohydrates from your diet, you must have a certain amount of natural carbohydrate for good health. Peas, beans, corn, and potatoes are about 15 to 20 percent carbohydrate and may have to be used sparingly on a reducing diet. They are not nearly as fattening as refined carbohydrates, however.

**4. Skimmed milk and skimmed milk products** such as cottage cheese and yogurt (for calcium and protein). If you cannot tolerate milk because of an inability to digest milk sugar or lactose, chances are you'll be able to handle *fermented* milk products all right. Most of the lactose in yogurt, for example, has been converted to lactic acid by bacterial action.

**5. Lean meat, skinned poultry, fish, eggs, and dried peas and beans** (for protein and B vitamins). Animal fat, in addition to being rich in calories, contains saturated fat and cholesterol that may be harmful to your arteries. So always cut away the fat from the meat you eat. Poultry and fish are low in harmful fat, and ocean fish supplies essential iodine. Try to get most of your protein from fish and poultry.

**6. Whole-grain bread, cereals, and flours** (for vitamin E and fiber). Always select *natural* whole-grain products that do not contain preservatives or additives. Rye and whole-wheat cereals, granola, oats, barley, and whole grits (not the quick-cooking variety), for example, supply fiber along with essential nutrients.

Do not use sugar on cereals! Use fresh or dried fruit instead.

**7. Vegetable oil or soft margarine** (for essential fatty acids). You must have some fat in your diet for good health. Cold-pressed vegetable oil is rich in the soft or unsaturated fat you need to keep animal fat from hardening in your arteries. Try to use about two tablespoons of vegetable oil (preferably safflower oil) on a green salad each day. Or use a *soft* margarine on whole-grain toast.


*Sunshine for Vitamin D*

Vitamin D is found primarily in fats of animal origin. Since skimmed milk and margarine are now enriched with vitamin D, you don't have to worry about a vitamin D deficiency on a low-fat diet that is properly balanced. Just to make sure that you get adequate vitamin D, however, and to keep your skin beautiful, follow the sunbathing instructions in chapter 6. You'll learn more in chapter 4 about how to balance your intake of vitamins.


**Beware of Specialized Diets**

Don't ever go on any kind of diet that restricts food selection to one type of food. In addition to resulting in a nutritional deficiency, a specialized diet can have other serious effects. A meat diet, for example, can trigger gouty arthritis, overload the kidneys, and contribute to the formation of kidney stones. (An excessive amount of phosphorus supplied by meat can result in urinary loss of calcium.) A fruit diet can result in loss of protein from muscles. A vegetable diet can contribute to development of anemia. A high-fat diet has been said to cause cancer or contribute to premature aging; it can also harden and clog arteries with a buildup of cholesterol and hard fat. Low carbohydrate diets that stress generous use of fats are so deficient in fiber that constipation becomes a serious problem. (For the best of health each day every woman needs a minimum of 60 to 100 grams of *natural* carbohydrate supplied by fruits, vegetables, and whole-grain products.)

So no matter what type of diet you follow to reduce your bodyweight, you should eat a *variety* of natural foods to protect your health. You need natural carbohydrate just as much as you need low-fat protein, and you need balanced amounts of all the essential nutrients. It's the *refined* carbohydrate that you don't need.

### How a Television Hostess Preserves Her Youthful Beauty

Helen Schuh, a former "Mrs. Ohio" who now hosts a television talk show, stays slim and youthful the celebrity way by avoiding refined carbohydrates. A specialist in female physical fitness, she first became fully aware of the value of natural foods in controlling bodyweight when she attended lectures at Peter Lupus Leisure Health World.

"When I gave up my exercise show on television, I found it more difficult to control my bodyweight since I was exercising less," she admitted. "But since going through Peter Lupus' program, I've learned to keep my weight down with proper selection of natural foods.

"Look at me!" she exclaimed recently as she stood before television cameras. "I eat nuts, cheese, and all kinds of goodies and I don't gain an ounce. I'm just as trim as I've ever been."

At 52 years of age, Helen Schuh is a mother of four, a promising actress, still beautiful, and still preparing for the future. Follow her example and preserve your health and your beauty so that you'll be ready for the best the future has to offer.

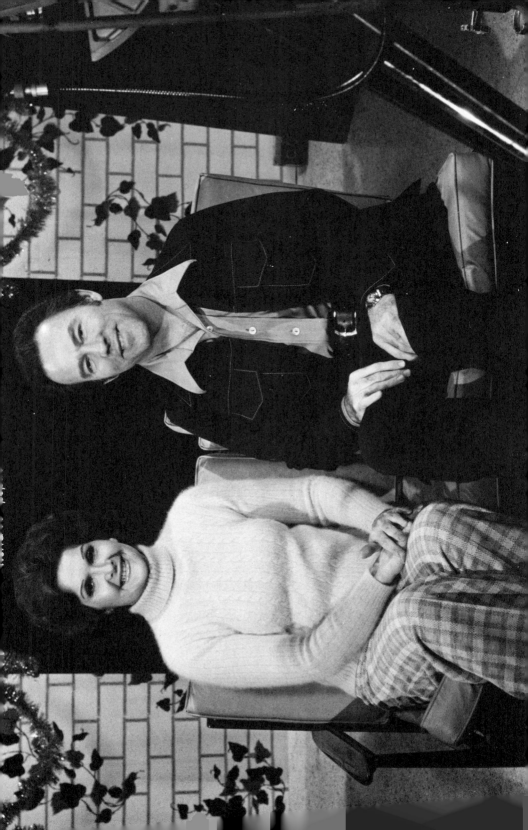

## Eight Basic Rules for Reducing Bodyweight
## with Natural Foods

If you are fairly active, as you should be, you can lose a few pounds a
week (and improve your health) simply by following a few basic rules.
1. Do not use sugar or eat foods containing sugar, white flour, or
   cornstarch.
2. Do not eat processed snacks of any kind.
3. Eat lean meats, skinned poultry, fish, eggs, fresh fruits and vegetables, raw salads, cottage cheese and yogurt made from
   skimmed milk, and whole-grain breads and cereals.
4. Use skimmed milk, unsweetened juices, and water as beverages.
   Drink *water* when you are thirsty!
5. Use two tablespoons of cold-pressed vegetable oil (such as
   safflower oil) on a green salad each day.
6. Eat slowly at mealtime. *Stop* eating when you feel comfortably
   satisfied.
7. Satisfy your craving for sweets by eating fresh and dried fruits for
   dessert following meals.
8. If you feel hungry, shaky, and weak between meals, eat a
   between-meal snack of baked chicken or a little yogurt or uncreamed cottage cheese with a piece of fresh fruit.

### A Sample Menu of Natural Foods

Since a natural foods diet for active people does not require counting
calories or measuring portions, a woman who exercises regularly can
follow a general diet plan successfully. It's not necessary to list specific
foods to be eaten at each meal if an effort is made to eat something from
all the basic food groups each day—or at least over a period of two days.
You can, in fact, pick the foods in each group that you like best. All you
have to do is make sure that your daily diet is balanced with fresh, natural
foods that have been properly prepared (see chapter 3). Your weight and
your appetite will automatically adjust at a level that is best for you.

Try these simple meal plans before considering the 1,200 calorie diet
outlined at the end of this chapter. Remember that none of the foods in
these plans should be cooked with grease or oil, and nothing should be
added except a little salt or bouillon (according to taste).

### Additional Hints for Dieters

If you feel that you need a snack between meals or at bedtime, try yogurt or uncreamed cottage cheese with fresh fruit. If you do have snacks between meals, you should eat *less* at mealtime.

Drink a few glasses of water between meals. Try to drink at least two glasses of skimmed milk or buttermilk each day.

Fish should be eaten as often as possible. Have liver at least once a week.

Add a little bran to your diet. Remember that bran taken with liquids provides considerable zero-calorie bulk.

---

### meal plans

*a breakfast plan*
One egg *or* a serving of lean ham, Canadian bacon, or veal.

One slice of whole-grain bread with a glass of skimmed milk *or* a whole-grain cereal with skimmed milk. (Raisins or diced fruit may be added to cereal.)

One piece of citrus fruit *or* a glass of fruit juice.

*a lunch plan*
Fish *or* skinned chicken *or* a lean meat of your choice. (Remember that chicken and fish are lowest in saturated fat.)

One dark-green *or* one deep-yellow vegetable.

One other vegetable of your choice.

One slice of whole-grain bread *or* a serving of coarse corn bread.

One glass of vegetable juice, water, *or* skimmed milk as a beverage with meal.

*For dessert*: melon, fresh fruit, *or* dried fruit. Unprocessed cheese with a serving of fresh fruit makes a satisfying dessert.

*a dinner plan*
A serving of the same meat dish you had at lunch *or* a serving of cottage cheese, pot cheese, or farmer cheese.

A fresh, raw vegetable salad laced with a tablespoon of cold-pressed vegetable oil.

A few whole-grain wafers or crackers.

A glass of juice or skimmed milk. (If you have fruit juice for breakfast, try to have vegetable juice for dinner.)

## a reducing diet for every woman

These recommended servings of basic foods, divided into three meals a day, supply about 1,200 calories.

Skimmed milk, 2 cups (1 pint) ......................176 calories

Egg, 1 medium..................................................81 calories

Lean meat, fish, or fowl,
4 ounces (cooked) .........................................376 calories

Vegetables (except potatoes)—2 servings of
yellow or deep green vegetables;
2 servings of other vegetables
(one-half cup each, cooked) ..........................144 calories

Fruit, citrus, 1 serving; other fruit,
2 servings.......................................................189 calories

Whole grain bread, 2 slices ...........................124 calories

Butter, margarine, or vegetable oil,
1 tablespoon (3 teaspoons) ..........................100 calories

Total number of calories: 1,190
Total grams of carbohydrate: 130

## 1200 calorie menu

*breakfast*
4 ounces orange juice
1 egg
1 slice whole-grain toast
1 teaspoon soft margarine
1 cup decaffeinated coffee (if desired)

*noon meal*
¼ cup uncreamed cottage cheese
Lettuce and tomato
1 slice whole-grain bread
1 teaspoon soft margarine
8 ounces skimmed milk
1 small apple

*evening meal*
3 ounces lean roast beef
½ cup beets
Cucumber and lettuce salad with vinegar and 1 teaspoon
    vegetable oil
8 ounces skimmed milk
2 medium dried apricots

## A Special 1200 Calorie Diet

If you're not very active and you find it difficult to lose weight on an unrestricted diet of natural foods, you can cut down your calorie intake by measuring food portions and limiting the size of your meals. But remember that you can do more for your body by exercising regularly so that you can eat generously. So be sure to try exercise and a general natural foods diet before resorting to calorie counting.

Most nutritionists maintain that you cannot get adequate amounts of all the essential nutrients on a diet containing less than 1,200 calories. It would be a good idea to take vitamin and mineral supplements with any low-calorie diet or a diet that results in a loss of more than two pounds a week.

Remember that a low-calorie diet might not be effective as a reducing diet if it includes small amounts of sugar and white-flour products. So be sure to stick to the recommended natural foods, with selections from the seven basic food groups.

### Adjust Your Diet According to Your Weight

When you begin to lose more than a couple of pounds a week, or when you want to cut down on further weight loss, start adding more raw salad, broiled fish, cottage cheese or yogurt, whole-grain cereals, and

---

**the modified 1200 calorie diet**

If you want to go on a temporary "crash" diet for a rapid weight loss, make these changes in the 1,200 calorie diet:

Reduce servings of vegetables to one serving of a deep-green or yellow vegetable.

Continue to eat one serving of citrus and reduce other fruits to only one serving.

Omit all bread.

Increase servings of meat, fish, or chicken from four ounces to seven ounces.

This will reduce the carbohydrate content of the diet to approximately 60 grams and increase your intake of iron and B vitamins. It's absolutely essential, however, that you take a multiple vitamin and mineral supplement while on such a diet.

other natural foods to your diet. You can adjust your food intake according to the amount of weight you are losing or gaining.

*Warning*: Remember that it's rarely necessary to go on a severely restricted diet if you exercise regularly. You should never stay on a diet that supplies fewer than 1,200 calories for more than a few weeks at a time.

### How a Fashion Model Lost 10 Pounds in 10 Days

Janet R., a beautiful, tall, fashion model, gained 10 pounds while on vacation in Europe. She wanted to lose 10 pounds in three weeks in order to accept an assignment modeling swimsuits. So she went on the modified 1,200 calorie diet and stepped up her exercise. She lost 10 pounds in 10 days! Janet didn't want her weight to go below 125 pounds, however, so she had to *increase* her intake of calories to prevent further weight loss. A little figuring revealed that she needed to take in at least 2,000 calories a day to keep her weight at the 125-pound level.

## How to Figure Your Calorie Requirement

When your weight is down where you want it, you may simply eat more to prevent further loss of weight. Or you may figure your calorie requirement exactly, as Janet did. Ordinarily, you would need 12 to 15 calories per pound of bodyweight each day to maintain your *existing* weight, depending upon how active you are. If you're inactive, you may need only about 12 calories per pound to maintain your weight. If you exercise regularly, however, you may need 15 or 16 calories for each pound of weight.

According to *Food and Your Weight*, published in 1973 by the U.S. Department of Agriculture, the average active woman needs about 16 calories each day for each pound of bodyweight. This means that a 125-pound woman would need about 2,000 calories each day to *maintain* her weight. (At least 200 additional calories would be needed during pregnancy, and as many as 1,000 additional calories during lactation.)

Weigh yourself about once a week to determine whether you're gaining or losing weight and then adjust your diet and your exercise accordingly. If you don't know how much you should weigh, stand nude before a mirror. If you don't appear to be fat, then you're not too fat.

If you want to count your calories to assure a weight loss, consult a food calorie chart so that you can select foods that will supply you with

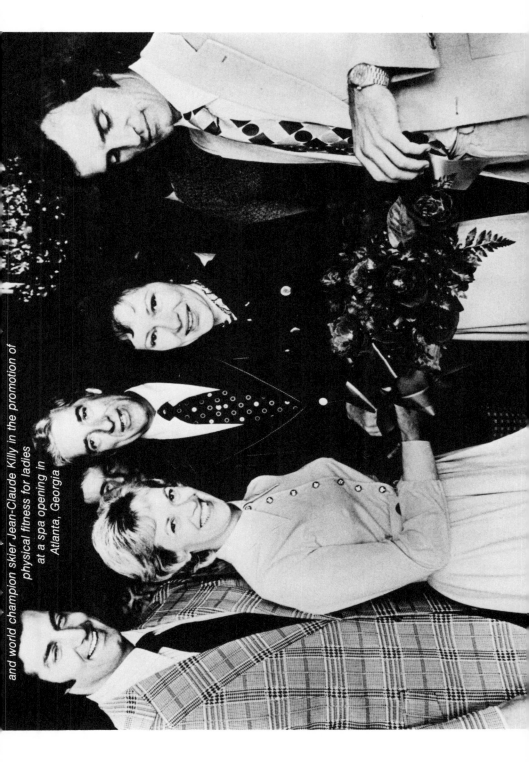

and world champion skier Jean-Claude Killy in the promotion of physical fitness for ladies at a spa opening in Atlanta, Georgia fewer calories than you would need to maintain your *existing* weight. Since there are about 3,500 calories in each pound of stored body fat, you can lose one pound a week for each 500-calorie deficit in your daily diet. Of course, the more exercise you take, the more calories you'll burn and the more weight you'll lose.

Since it's difficult to measure calorie intake and output accurately, calorie counting is not very practical. Simply cutting down on food intake and taking more exercise will usually do the trick. If you'd like to learn more about reducing your bodyweight and counting calories, read *Doctor Homola's Fat-Disintegrator Diet* (Parker Publishing Company).

### Fat and Female Shapeliness

In your zeal to reduce your bodyweight, don't get too thin! You need a little body fat in reserve to meet medical emergencies. Besides, most men prefer their women to have soft, cuddly curves.

Ask your man how he likes you best. There's no sense in knocking yourself out to lose those last few pounds, or those "love handles," if your man likes you the way you are.

## SUMMARY

1. Any overweight woman can lose weight simply by eliminating sugar and refined carbohydrates from her diet.

2. Overweight women who have a blood sugar problem must avoid refined carbohydrates, coffee, tea, and colas, and eat a high-protein snack between meals.

3. Women who exercise regularly can eat generous amounts of properly prepared natural foods and still lose weight.

4. Adding bran or fiber to the diet will help reduce bodyweight as well as help prevent diseases of the intestinal tract.

5. Each day every woman should try to eat food selections from the seven basic food groups.

6. Women who are not physically active can lose weight on a special 1,200 calorie diet that includes food selections from all the basic food groups.

7. Specialized diets that restrict food selections to one type of food can result in development of disease or illness.

8. Your weight and your appetite will automatically adjust on a general diet of natural foods, but you must periodically adjust a low-calorie diet.

9. Don't try to get rid of all the fat on your body. Remember that the beauty of your body will depend largely upon natural feminine fat molded by well-developed muscles.

10. No matter what type of diet you follow, foods must be properly prepared for maximum nutrients with minimum calories, so be sure to read chapter 3.

# simple ways to prepare healthful, body-slimming foods

Since the foods you eat have more to do with your health and your physical appearance than any other single factor, it's very important that your foods be properly prepared. This doesn't mean that you have to be a gourmet cook who prepares fancy dishes. It means that you must use *simple cooking methods* to conserve nutrients. Remember that you must eat to keep your body healthy as well as beautiful. So it's important to keep nutrients up and calories down.

The cooking hints in this chapter cannot compete with the culinary skills of the beautiful ladies reading this book. What you learn in reading this chapter, however, will encourage you to place health before taste when preparing foods. Luckily, natural foods prepared in a simple way actually taste *better* than foods that have been overcooked and dressed up with sauces, and they have fewer calories.

Once you have tried simple cooking methods and experienced the tasty, original flavors of basic, natural foods, chances are you'll give up complicated cooking methods that destroy nutrients and disguise the true taste of food.

### Basic Guidelines for Preparing Basic Foods

Since the heart of a good nutritional program is based upon use of the seven basic food groups, all you have to do to eat properly is to learn

54

# *Chapter 3*

how to prepare the basic foods. In many cases, there isn't even any cooking to do. All fruits and some vegetables are more nutritious when eaten raw. When a vegetable does need cooking, a little steaming may be all that's necessary. Cooking for health is very simple. Eating for health can be a pleasure. Don't complicate it all with strange and exotic cooking methods. Remember that simplicity is the key to good health when it comes to eating.

Every woman, whether she is a movie star or a housewife, can use the same basic guidelines in preparing and eating foods. In fact, the authors of this book are offering to you the same advice they offer to glamorous stars and celebrities who *must* look good and feel good to withstand the rigors and the competition of stardom.

## Charo—a Dynamo of Energy!

If you watch television, you've seen Charo perform. This blonde, beautiful bundle of energy has appeared as a guest on *all* the TV game and talk shows and was recently featured in her own TV special. She is one of Hollywood's fastest rising stars—and the most energetic.

In addition to her TV work, she is a frequent headliner in Las Vegas. She spends at least four hours a day singing and

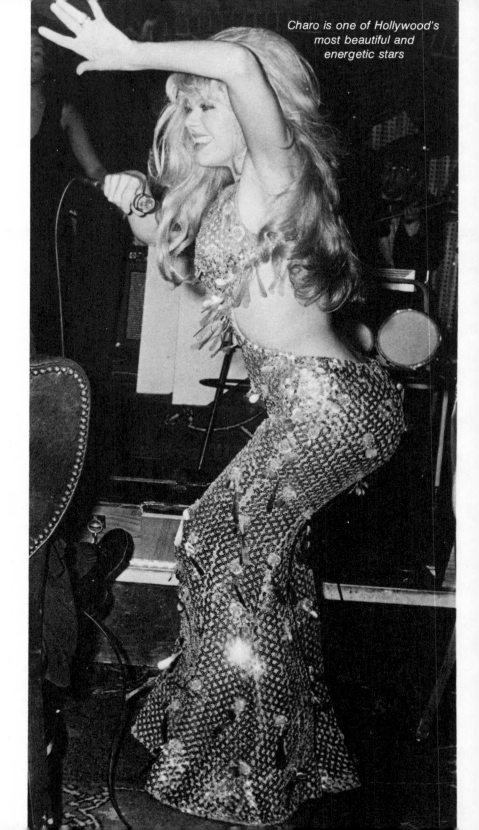

Charo is one of Hollywood's most beautiful and energetic stars practicing with her guitar. She swims and does dance exercises *every day*, and she goes disco dancing twice a week! How does she do all this and still manage to remain so fresh and energetic? Good nutrition is part of the answer.

Charo includes such basic foods as cheese, fresh fruit, and seafood in her diet. Her favorite food is a Spanish dish that contains rice, lobster, shrimp, and various other seafoods. "I also include saffron herbs to help make me sexy," she confessed. "I use a special herb tea from Spain as a pickup. And I make sure that I get at least five or six hours of sleep each night."

No one has more energy than Charo. Her health habits obviously work well for her. With all her beauty, talent, energy, and good health, she cannot fail in her climb to stardom.

No matter what you do in life, you must be healthy and energetic to succeed. You certainly must be healthy to be happy!

### A Nutritional Deficiency Can Kill You

You *are* what you eat. A nutritional deficiency will make itself apparent in your physical appearance as well as in your performance. It can also kill you! According to *Human Nutrition*, published by the U.S. Department of Agriculture, "Most of the health problems underlying the leading causes of death in the United States could be modified by improvements in diet."

### Eat Different to Be Different

In years past, the use of vitamins, natural foods, and organically grown fruits and vegetables has been looked upon as faddism. Today, however, it is becoming increasingly more evident that the *real* faddists are not those who take vitamins and eat natural foods, but those who blindly gulp down refined and artificial foods. So don't give up your preference for properly prepared natural foods just because someone criticizes your diet.

It is now well known that the standard American diet is responsible for most of the nation's major health problems. If you want to be radiantly healthy, beautiful, and energetic, you shouldn't eat like the average American. You should eat *better*! And this means careful attention to selecting and preparing your foods properly.

*Carol Channing*, one of Broadway's most popular and energetic stars, keeps her energy up with a special diet of properly prepared natural foods. "I believe in doing things the natural way whenever possible," she said in a *Family Health* interview. "I eat only organic foods that have been grown without any chemical fertilizer or artificial growth stimulant."

*Hildegarde*, whose singing has thrilled the world for more than 50 years, supplements a low-calorie natural foods diet with vitamins. "There are those who think of me as a food faddist," she revealed recently in a published interview, "but what I am is a woman past her middle years whose way of earning a living demands she look well and possess above-average energy."

### The Health Secrets of Aniko Farrell, "Miss Canada"

We all fell in love with Aniko Farrell when she visited Peter Lupus Leisure Health World. This lovely singer and actress, a former "Miss Canada" and a first runner-up "Miss World," now the wife of actor Peter Palmer, has a warm smile and a friendly manner that make her absolutely irresistible.

Aniko is also radiantly healthy and beautiful, and she attributes her good health to good eating habits. "Peter and I eat lots of fruit," she replied to a question about her diet, "and we *steam* all our fresh vegetables. We eat lots of chicken and fish. And we supplement our diet with vitamin $B_{12}$, vitamin C, iron, lecithin, kelp, and calcium lactate. When we're doing a show, we take plenty of extra vitamin C to make sure that we don't catch a cold. And believe me, it works! We cannot afford to get sick because there are no understudies in summer stock."

Since Aniko and her husband are both very active in television and on the stage, neither can afford illness or poor health. Both have starred *together* in a great number of stage hits, such as "Li'l Abner," "My Fair Lady," and "The Sound of Music." More recently, they co-starred with Carol Channing in the hit Broadway musical "Lorelei."

Like Carol Channing, Aniko must pay close attention to her health habits in order to withstand a busy and hectic schedule of singing, dancing, and acting. In addition to eating properly, Aniko stays physically fit by doing the Canadian Air Force exercises every day for 15 minutes.

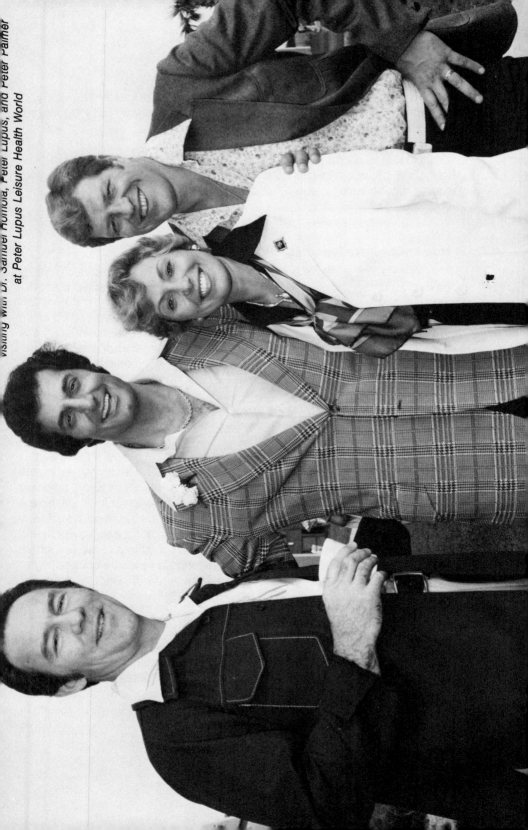

visiting with Dr. Samuel Homola, Peter Lupus, and Peter Palmer at Peter Lupus Leisure Health World

Whatever *your* role in life might be, housewife or career woman, you, too, must stay healthy and fit if you want to avoid incapacitating illness. Chances are, there are no understudies who can replace *you* if you get sick.

How you *prepare* your foods can be just as important as proper selection of foods in getting the nutrients you need to preserve your health. So be sure to study this chapter carefully.

### How to Conserve Nutrients in Vegetables

Vegetables suffer more from improper cooking methods than any other type of food. The carbohydrate in vegetables is unaffected by cooking, but many of the essential vitamins are washed out by water or destroyed by heat, light, and air. The cellulose in vegetables, which is so important for good bowel health, may also lose its effectiveness if it is overcooked. This means that if you cook vegetables improperly, you may have nothing left but carbohydrate that supplies calories without nutrients. We all know that empty calories build up fat while tearing down health.

You should eat vegetables *raw* whenever possible. When vegetables are cooked, they should be cooked as little as possible.

The best way to be assured of getting a maximum amount of nutrients from vegetables is to eat a *raw* salad each day. And, in addition to the usual lettuce and tomatoes, you should include a wide variety of raw vegetables. Any vegetable that is edible can be eaten raw. Every time you cook a vegetable, put some aside for use in a raw salad. Or simply take a few bites. Don't try to eat all of your vegetables raw, however. Many vegetables, such as carrots, spinach, broccoli, and cauliflower, yield more nutrients when they have been cooked a little. So while certain vegetables, such as lettuce and tomatoes, should never be cooked, other vegetables should be eaten both ways—raw and cooked.

### *How to Cook Fresh Vegetables*

You can best conserve the taste and the nutrients in any vegetable by cooking it in the shortest time possible with as little heat as possible. Generous use of water in cooking shortens cooking time but increases loss of nutrients. Cooking without water in "waterless cookware" results in loss of nutrients by prolonging exposure to heat.

## A Simple Technique for Steaming a Vegetable

Probably the best way to cook a vegetable is to put just enough water in the pot to prevent scorching and then cook the vegetable on low heat long enough to soften it a little. Be sure to use a pot with a tight-fitting lid so that steam from the water will displace air and aid in cooking. When the vegetable is tender enough to penetrate with a fork, it is cooked enough. A cooked vegetable that is still crisp has more taste as well as more nutrients. Never cook a vegetable until it is soft and mushy.

If there is any water left in the pot after cooking a vegetable, be sure to use the water as a soup or a beverage. Water from cooked vegetables is loaded with water-soluble vitamins and minerals.

You can also steam a vegetable by placing it in a covered perforated pan or colander that is resting over a pot of boiling water. The steam passing up through the vegetables will do the cooking without washing out nutrients. Just make sure that the vegetable does not come in contact with the water.

*Note*: Don't salt your vegetables until *after* they have been cooked, preferably just before serving. Salt may draw nutrients from the vegetables, draining them into the bottom of the pot.

You should always cook vegetables without adding grease or oil. Properly cooked vegetables are delicious without using fat as a seasoning. Besides, you don't need the calories supplied by greasy vegetables. You'll get all the fat you need from lean meats and from a few tablespoons of vegetable oil daily on a green salad.

## Cutting and Peeling Vegetables

Don't peel a raw vegetable that has an edible skin. You need the fiber and the nutrients supplied by every part of the vegetable. Remember that fiber supplies low-calorie bulk that will help keep you slim.

When you cook vegetables, cut them into pieces just large enough to permit cooking. The more of the vegetable that's exposed to light and air, the greater the loss of nutrients. You should *never* shred a vegetable.

When you boil root or tubular vegetables, such as carrots and small potatoes, do not peel or cut them unless you have to. If the skin of a vegetable is intact, you can boil it with very little or no loss of nutrients.

## What About Potatoes?

The best way to cook potatoes is to *bake* them in their skin.

You can make a nonfattening imitation sour cream for your potatoes by mixing two-thirds cup cottage cheese with one-fourth cup buttermilk and one-half teaspoon lemon juice. Mix in a blender and chill in a refrigerator before serving.

If some members of your family refuse to eat the jacket of a baked potato, scoop out the potato and put the shell back in the oven for about five minutes. A potato jacket browned in this manner, seasoned with a little salt, is delicious.

### How to Boil Frozen Vegetables

Although steaming is the best way to cook fresh vegetables, you may have to boil frozen vegetables to prevent loss of nutrients during thawing.

Put enough water into a pot to equal about one-third of the volume of the vegetables you want to cook. Bring the water to a boil and then drop in the frozen vegetables. Cover the pot with a lid and cook just long enough to soften the vegetables. Remember that frozen vegetables are partially cooked during the blanching process that precedes freezing, so they won't require as much cooking as raw vegetables.

### Beware of Leftovers

It's always best to cook your vegetables *fresh* each day. Leftover vegetables lose nutrients, especially vitamin C, when they are refrigerated and then reheated. They also lose taste. Cook just enough vegetables for *one day*. Serve them immediately after cooking. Keep leftover vegetables covered between meals to prevent exposure to air and light.

Fresh vegetables are so simple to prepare that your effort in preparing them each day is a small price to pay for the nutrients they supply. If you don't have time to cook your vegetables, eat them raw rather than do without them or eat day-old leftovers.

Many celebrities who have a traveling schedule that does not permit much time for cooking choose to carry fresh, raw vegetables with them wherever they go. Snacking on raw vegetables gives them the fiber and the nutrients they need to maintain good health with normal bowel function.

### Fruits Should Always Be Eaten Raw

Fruits are delicious as well as nutritious when eaten raw. You should *never* cook a fruit when you can eat it raw. And you should always eat the *whole fruit* rather than squeeze it for juice.

*Special note:* Fruit juice is sometimes helpful in relieving the pain of cystitis. The urine is normally acid, but when the bladder and the urethra are so raw and inflamed that urination causes a burning pain, drinking a large amount of fruit and vegetable juice will help relieve the pain by *alkalizing* the urine. Cranberries and plums are the only fresh fruits that add acid to the urine. Cranberry juice may be helpful in *preventing* infection in a healthy bladder, since bacteria normally do not multiply in an acid environment.

### Whole Fruit Has Special Value

When the skin of a fruit is edible, wash the fruit and eat it whole. Both the skin and the pulp of fresh, raw fruit supply nutrients as well as healthful bulk for your bowels.

Fruits contain a variety of vitamins and minerals, but they are best known as a valuable source of vitamin C. In addition to its role in protecting your health, the ascorbic acid (vitamin C) supplied by fruits aids your stomach in absorbing iron and calcium. Citrus fruits are the best sources of ascorbic acid.

Yellow fruits, such as apricots, peaches, cantaloupes, mangoes, and papayas, are fairly good sources of vitamin A. Fruits also contain enzymes that might be beneficial to health. Pineapple and papaya, for example, contain enzymes that can aid your stomach in the digestion of protein.

Strawberries compare favorably with citrus fruit as a source of vitamin C. A few other berries are also rich in vitamin C. But since citrus fruits are our most readily available source of this vitamin, you should try to eat at least one serving of citrus fruit every day. Every woman needs a citrus fruit and a dark-green or deep-yellow vegetable each day along with two additional servings of fruits or vegetables.

### Do You Get Enough Vitamin C?

One orange supplies about 25 milligrams of vitamin C. You must have at least 70 milligrams of vitamin C each day to prevent the development of disease. Raw cabbage, tomatoes, and other vegetables, even potatoes, supply vitamin C, so you don't have to depend entirely upon fruit as your source. But just to make sure that you get enough vitamin C for radiant health, try to get your daily quota from fresh fruits and then get all the additional vitamin C you can from properly prepared vegetables.

Some nutritionists feel that most of us need much more vitamin C than the recommended daily allowance proposed for the "average" person. So the more fruit you eat, the better. Be sure to study the material on vitamin C in chapter 4.

*Note:* You need only about 10 milligrams of vitamin C each day to prevent scurvy. But less than the recommended daily allowance of vitamin C may contribute to the development of other diseases.

### Fruits Won't Make You Fat

Don't worry about your weight or your blood sugar when you eat fresh fruit. Fructose, or fruit sugar, is not as fattening as refined sugar and it won't overload your pancreas. Since fruit is low in sodium, it won't have any adverse effects on your blood pressure, either.

The pectin in fruit helps detoxify your body by absorbing toxins from your intestinal tract and by aiding bowel function. There's no reason why you can't eat all the fruit you want, even if you don't feel that you need additional vitamin C.

### How to Use Skimmed Milk and Skimmed Milk Products

Even if you're not overweight or having trouble with the cholesterol or triglyceride levels in your blood, you should go easy on your consumption of milk fat. You'll get all the fat you need from meats and vegetable oil. You don't need the calories and the hard fat supplied by whole milk. So, as a matter of prevention, it's best to depend upon *skimmed milk* and its products for calcium, protein, and B vitamins.

Milk loses riboflavin (vitamin $B_2$) when exposed to light. Make sure that your milk is protected from sunlight, daylight, or artificial light. If your milkman leaves milk on your back porch every morning, it should be in an opaque container.

Don't use nondairy creamers. They usually contain coconut oil, which is a saturated fat, and they are loaded with artificial additives.

The best way to get all the nutritional benefits of milk is to drink skimmed milk as a beverage with meals. Or you may use milk with whole-grain cereals or in other appropriate dishes. Remember, however, that when you remove the fat from milk you also remove the vitamin A. So if you use skimmed milk, you should eat more yellow vegetables or use a *fortified* soft margarine.

*What to Substitute if Milk Upsets Your Stomach*

Unfortunately, many adults do not have the intestinal enzyme they need to digest lactose (milk sugar). As a result, when they drink fresh milk they suffer from diarrhea, cramps, and other symptoms of indigestion. If you cannot tolerate milk, chances are you can handle *fermented* milk products. When milk is fermented to produce yogurt, buttermilk, cottage cheese, pot cheese, or farmer's cheese, most of the lactose in the milk is converted to lactic acid by bacterial action.

Fermented milk products are just as rich in calcium and protein as fresh milk, but some of the B vitamins, especially $B_{12}$, may be lost in the fermentation process. Other animal and dairy products in your diet, however, will supply adequate amounts of vitamin $B_{12}$.

*Yogurt Aids Intestinal Function*

Since yogurt supplies a friendly bacteria that combats the harmful bacteria in your colon, you should include yogurt in your diet, even if you drink skimmed milk. To avoid artificial additives, buy your yogurt in a health food store or simply make your own.

### how to make yogurt

Heat a quart of milk to the boiling point to kill undesirable bacteria. Cool the milk to a temperature of about 100 degrees Fahrenheit. Then add a lactobacillus culture (preferably acidophilus) or a heaping tablespoon of fresh plain yogurt to the milk and stir well. Pour the milk into six small glass containers with lids. Keep the milk heated to a temperature of about 110 degrees until it thickens, which will take several hours. Then place the newly made yogurt in the refrigerator.

*Note*: During the process of making yogurt, if the temperature of the milk is kept below 90 degrees or above 120 degrees Fahrenheit, the milk may not congeal properly. If the fermentation process is allowed to continue after the milk has congealed, the yogurt may become watery.

To get the best-tasting yogurt possible, purchase yogurt culture and a yogurt maker at your local health food store or department store. With this appliance you will be able to control the temperature and the time exactly.

### How to Prepare Lean Meats, Poultry, Fish, Eggs, and Dried Peas and Beans

The foods in this group are eaten primarily for the protein they supply. If you don't eat meat, you can get adequate protein from poultry, fish, eggs, or dairy products. Peas and beans are good sources of protein, but, with the exception of soybeans, they do not contain a *complete* protein. When peas or beans are substituted for meat, fish, or poultry in a balanced diet, however, your body combines protein from the different sources to form a complete protein.

### *Meat Fat Is Bad for You*

When you prepare meat of any kind, you should *cut away all the visible fat before cooking the meat*. Remember that meat fat contains cholesterol and saturated fats that tend to harden and clog arteries. Your female hormones help protect you against the onset of hardened arteries until after menopause. But since animal fat adds weight to your body and may contribute to the development of colon cancer, the less fat you eat the better.

### *Broiled Fish Is Best*

It's usually best to roast, bake, or broil your meats on a rack so that fat dripping from the meat can be collected in the bottom of the pan for disposal.

Chicken and fish should also be baked or broiled. Just remember not to eat the chicken skin. And be careful not to overcook your fish. It takes only a few minutes to cook fish. When the flesh of fish changes from a transparent color to creamy white and is easily flaked with a fork, it is done enough to eat. Since fish is low in fat and calories, you can eat as much of it as you want—as long as it is not fried or cooked in oil or fat.

If you're not particularly fond of fish, you may poach it or steam it for use in a salad.

Try to eat *ocean* fish so that your thyroid gland will get the iodine it needs to control your bodyweight. If you eat plenty of seafood, you won't have to depend upon table salt for iodine. And the less salt you use, the easier it is to shed excess weight.

## Eggs Are Good for You

If you're not having trouble with high blood cholesterol, there's no reason why you cannot eat an egg or two every day. In addition to being a good source of protein, whole eggs supply vitamin A and other nutrients that tend to be deficient in a low-fat diet. The essential fatty acids in egg yolk tend to counteract the cholesterol in the yolk. Just be careful not to destroy the fatty acids by overcooking the egg. Soft-boiled eggs are best. You can also scramble or poach an egg without overheating the yolk.

## Be Careful with Peas and Beans

Fresh peas and beans may be cooked simply by boiling them in a little water. But when you cook *dried* peas and beans, you must use a different cooking method to conserve nutrients. When you cook dried beans, for example, first drop the beans into a pot of boiling water and cook them for two minutes. Then remove the pot from the stove and let the beans soak in the cooking water for one hour before finishing the cooking. This will eliminate the customary 15 hours of cold-water soaking. It also permits you to use the soaking water as cooking water, thus retaining all the water-soluble vitamins and minerals.

## Soybeans Are Special

Since the soybean is the only vegetable that can supply a complete protein equivalent to meat, you might want to eat soybeans occasionally as a meat substitute. Remember, however, that if you do not eat meat, you

---

### how to boil soybeans

Place a cup or two of dried soybeans in a bowl of cold water and let them soak overnight. Remember that the dried beans will increase in size when they absorb water, so be sure to use a large bowl. Cover the beans with water, leaving two or three inches of water above the beans.

When you are ready to cook the beans, place the soaking water and the beans in a heavy kettle. If necessary, add enough extra water to cover the beans. Throw in a pinch of salt, bring the water to a boil, and then simmer over low heat for three or four hours until the beans are tender.

should include eggs or dairy products in your diet for the vitamin $B_{12}$ you need to build healthy blood cells.

There are many ways to cook soybeans to alter their taste. For example, they may be cooked in soup stock, with tomato sauce, or in a casserole. You can even make patties that are as delicious as hamburger. Look for a good cookbook that tells you how to prepare soybeans in a variety of ways. In the meantime, the simplest way to cook soybeans is to boil them.

### How to Use Whole-Grain Breads, Cereals, and Flours

Whole-grain products are good sources of vitamin E. They also supply bran, or fiber, which is essential for good bowel health. To keep your diet balanced, eat a whole-grain product each day in addition to the whole-grain bread you have with your meals. You don't have to worry too much about the calories in whole-grain products if they are coarse and

---

#### how to make high-fiber whole-grain bread

If you make your own bread (it's easy!), you can use rye, whole-wheat, or whatever type of flour you prefer. Here's a recipe for bran-rich whole-wheat bread:

Mix 3 cups warm water with ½ cup honey and 2 packages baker's yeast. Allow this mixture to stand for 5 minutes or longer and then add 4½ cups unsifted stone-ground whole-wheat flour and ½ cup pure bran. Beat this mixture by hand 100 times or more.

Then add 2 or 3 cups more whole-wheat flour (or enough to make the dough stiff) and 1 scant tablespoon salt.

Knead the dough until it is smooth and elastic, adding enough flour to prevent sticking.

Place the dough in an oiled bowl, and let sit in a warm place until the dough rises to double in bulk.

Knead the dough back to its original size and place it in two 1½-pound loaf pans that have been greased with margarine.

Let the dough rise until it reaches the top of the pan before placing it in the oven.

Bake in a preheated oven at 350 degrees for about 60 minutes or until the bread is well browned.

completely natural. If you add additional bran, as suggested in chapter 2, whole-grain products will actually aid in reducing your bodyweight.

### *Cereals Should Be Unprocessed*

There are many natural whole-grain cereals on the shelves of grocery stores and health food stores. No special preparation is needed. Just make sure that you don't pick up a processed or quick-cooking cereal. Whenever possible, buy the ready-to-eat unsweetened variety and use fresh or dried fruit rather than sugar as a sweetener. Shredded wheat is a good basic cereal. So is granola.

### How to Use Vegetable Oil and Margarine

There's nothing wrong with eating a little butter occasionally, since it supplies vitamins A and D and other essential nutrients. Too much butter, however, may contribute to a buildup of cholesterol in your blood, so it's best to depend upon vegetable oil for essential fatty acids. Remember, however, that all fats and oils are high in calories. A few tablespoons of vegetable oil daily on a green salad or a little soft margarine on whole-grain breakfast toast will give you all the fat you need in a balanced diet.

Although margarine is made of vegetable oil, a *hard* margarine may be just as harmful to your arteries as butter or animal fat. When vegetable oil has been hardened by a process called "hydrogenation," the essential fatty acids in the oil are converted to hard (saturated) fat. A margarine that is soft, however, or only partially hydrogenated, contains a higher percentage of essential fatty acids.

You can add healthful, essential fatty acids to margarine by mixing in a little safflower oil. Just be careful not to add so much oil that the refrigerated margarine will be too liquid to spread on toast.

### *Heat Damages Essential Fatty Acids*

If you must watch the calories in your diet, you should not eat fried foods. Cooking with fat or oil adds extra calories. When you do need to use fat or oil in cooking, you should use vegetable oil. In addition to supplying essential fatty acids, vegetable oil has a higher smoking temperature than animal fat and can therefore withstand higher temperatures. When you heat vegetable oil to temperatures above 419 degrees

Fahrenheit (215 degrees Centigrade) for 15 minutes or longer, however, the fatty acids begin to smoke and break down into a toxic substance that can irritate your intestinal tract. So don't try to depend upon heated oils for your essential fatty acids, and never heat cooking fats or oils until they begin to smoke.

If you use a few tablespoons of cold-pressed vegetable oil on a green salad each day, or if you use enriched soft margarine on toast, you can do without fats and oils in cooking.

## SUMMARY

1. The basic natural foods prepared in the simplest manner possible will supply the nutrients you need to be healthy and beautiful.

2. When you cook vegetables, use as little heat, water, and time as possible. Steaming is best!

3. Eat raw salads often, and include a variety of *raw vegetables* in the salads whenever possible.

4. Cook your vegetables *fresh* every day, so that you won't have to eat vitamin-depleted leftovers.

5. You can eat a variety of fresh fruits without gaining weight—providing you eat them *raw*.

6. The pain of cystitis (inflamed urinary bladder) can sometimes be relieved by alkalizing the urine with fruit and vegetable juices.

7. If fresh milk upsets your stomach, try using *fermented* milk products, such as yogurt, made of skimmed milk.

8. Broiled fish is a better and safer source of low-fat protein than meats and eggs.

9. If you make homemade bread, use a whole-grain flour that you have enriched with bran.

10. If you use margarine, stir in a little safflower oil to enrich the margarine with essential fatty acids.

# vitamins and minerals work miracles with your health

If your diet is balanced with basic natural foods that have been properly prepared, chances are you'll get all the nutrients you need to maintain good health. But if your health is poor, or if you have been eating improperly for many years, you may need additional amounts of certain vitamins and minerals to restore your health. In other words, you may need *megavitamin therapy*.

Once a vitamin or mineral deficiency appears, your body no longer has any reserve amounts of that particular nutrient. And when there is a deficiency in one vitamin or mineral, there is usually also a deficiency in other nutrients. Before you can be radiantly healthy and beautiful, you must reach the point where you are taking enough of the essential vitamins and minerals to maintain reserves.

You'll learn in this chapter how to recognize the symptoms of nutritional deficiencies and how to correct them. Every woman can benefit from the use of certain vitamin and mineral supplements. Even when your diet is adequate, uncontrollable factors may create a need for additional amounts of certain nutrients. No two women have exactly the same nutritional needs. Some need more or less of certain nutrients. If you're under a great deal of stress, for example, you may need more vitamin C than the "average" woman. So don't assume that just because you get the recommended daily allowances of the basic nutrients you're getting all you need. You must go by the way you feel. If you don't feel well, you might be able to help yourself by supplementing your diet. Correcting a nutritional deficiency can result in miraculous changes in your health and your physical appearance.

# *Chapter 4*

How Judy Made Miraculous Changes in Her Health

Judy B. complained of not feeling well. "I just don't have any energy," she related. "I'm so nervous all the time I'm constantly suffering from indigestion. Besides that, I don't sleep well at night. All the doctors I've been to say there's nothing wrong with me. I'm getting very depressed. Do you think I'm a hypochondriac?"

One look at Judy's physical appearance revealed a possible cause for *all* her complaints: nutritional deficiency. Her skin was dry and goose-bumpy. There were tiny red cracks in the corners of her mouth. She was obviously losing hair, and her fingernails were pale and rough.

Judy admitted that her diet left a lot to be desired. "I've been working part time," she confessed, "and going to school to complete my studies for my master's degree. I haven't been eating much except diet colas and hamburgers."

Judy was so nutritionally deficient that she had to take food supplements to restore her vitamin and mineral reserves. The results were dramatic. Her nervous and digestive symptoms were relieved almost immediately. All of the symptoms that had plagued her for years were cleared up in a few weeks. Judy went on to complete her studies with vigor. And in her spare time she began an earnest study of nutrition.

If you have been eating improperly and have developed a nutritional deficiency, you, too, can get miraculous results from food supplements. Study the material in this chapter to determine if you might need additional amounts of any particular vitamin or mineral. Make sure, however, that you improve your diet in order to correct the *cause* of your nutritional deficiency.

---

### Suzanne Somers—Actress, Author, and Gourmet Chef!

Tall, blonde, and blue-eyed Suzanne Somers, who stars in the ABC hit comedy series "Three's Company," keeps herself physically beautiful by eating properly, taking vitamins and minerals, and exercising with a barbell. A gourmet chef who has actually *taught* cooking, Suzanne prepares her own meals to make sure that her intake of sugar, salt, and fat will not be too high. Chicken is her favorite "meat," and she prepares it often with vegetables and herbs taken from her own organically grown garden.

Although secure in an acting career that includes many movie, television, and stage credits, Suzanne's varied talents continue to burst out in all directions. Already the author of two best-selling books of poetry, she has authored a third book entitled *Some People Live More than Others*. She also hopes to write a cookbook and sing in a Broadway musical. She has no doubt that she'll eventually accomplish these objectives.

"I firmly believe that you can do anything you want to do if you plant the seed," she explains. "There's an area in our subconscious that responds to our dreams and desires if we sincerely direct our energies to it."

---

Remember that no matter what *your* goals might be, you'll have to be healthy to reach them and enjoy them. Suzanne Somers, like all beautiful, successful women, makes self-help health care a part of her way of life in order to assure success in her endeavors. "You can do anything you want to do if you maximize your potential," she advises. Needless to say, your potential depends as much upon your health as upon your beauty and your talent.

### How to Get the Nutrients You Need Most

There are about 40 nutrients known to be vital in human nutrition. If you make an effort to eat foods containing certain essential vitamins and

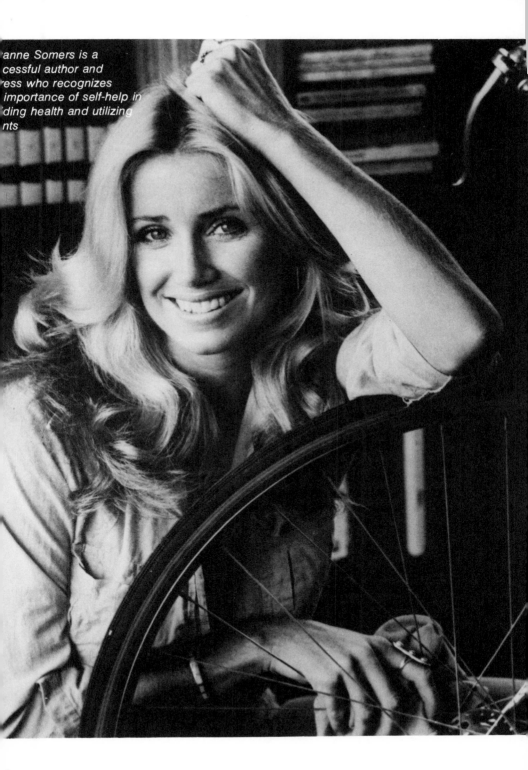

anne Somers is a
cessful author and
ress who recognizes
importance of self-help in
ding health and utilizing
nts

minerals, you'll automatically get all the other vital nutrients. For example, if your diet supplies vitamins A, B, C, D, and E, and the minerals calcium, phosphorus, iron, and iodine, and your diet is balanced with the basic natural foods to supply adequate amounts of protein, carbohydrate, and fat (as recommended in chapter 2), chances are you'll get adequate amounts of all the other vital nutrients. If your body is diseased, however, deficiencies may develop that are difficult or impossible to correct with food supplements. In the case of pernicious anemia, for example, inability of the stomach to absorb vitamin $B_{12}$ may make it necessary for a physician to *inject* the vitamin in order to control the disease. Diseases of the intestinal tract may interfere with absorption of certain nutrients, and so on. When you are ill, or when you present symptoms of disease, be sure to see a physician for diagnosis and treatment. In the meantime, your own efforts in making sure that your body gets adequate amounts of the essential nutrients can make the difference between being radiantly healthy or dull, lifeless, and tired.

### Slight Deficiencies Are Difficult to Detect

Many of us suffer from subclinical nutritional deficiencies, which means that we are deficient enough to look and feel unwell, but not deficient enough to present classical symptoms of disease. Any doctor can recognize the obvious symptoms of a severe vitamin deficiency, as in scurvy or pellagra, but few will recognize symptoms caused by subclinical deficiencies. You don't have to wait until you are obviously ill to take a vitamin or mineral supplement for a *suspected* deficiency. You can help yourself safely and effectively with foods *and* supplements.

### Vitamin A for Healthy, Beautiful Skin

Vitamin A is best known for its role in preventing night blindness and diseases of the eye. It's also essential for healthy skin and in helping the body resist infection. The membranes that line the inside of glands and organs, as in bronchial tubes, sinuses, the throat, and the bladder, are particularly susceptible to chronic infection when vitamin A stores are low or depleted. So, if you suffer from bronchitis, sinusitis, cystitis, or any chronic problem involving the membranes and the skin of your body, a vitamin A supplement might help.

The best sources of vitamin A are liver, egg yolk, butter, cream, fortified margarine, and dark-green or yellow vegetables. *Liver is the richest source of vitamin A.* Unfortunately, animal products containing vitamin A are also rich in saturated fat or cholesterol. The carotene in yellow or dark-green vegetables can be converted to vitamin A by the body. Persons on a low-fat diet may tend to be deficient in vitamin A and once the symptoms of a deficiency appear, it may be necessary to take a vitamin A supplement, such as fish liver oil. If you cannot tolerate oil, you can purchase vitamin A in water-soluble tablet form.

*Note:* Dryness and scaliness of the skin, sometimes with hardened goose bumps, is an *early* sign of vitamin A deficiency.

### How to Use Supplements to Correct a
### Vitamin A Deficiency

For adults the recommended daily allowance of vitamin A is 5,000 units (6,000 if you are pregnant and 8,000 if you are breast feeding). Some nutritionists believe that up to 25,000 units may be needed daily for the best of health and for a long life. Yet, a nationwide survey of household food consumption in 1965 indicated that 27 percent of all households consumed diets that supplied *less* than 5,000 units!

When you suspect that you are suffering from a vitamin A deficiency, you should take from 25,000 to 35,000 units a day for a few months. Since vitamin A is a fat-soluble vitamin that can be stored in the body, an excessive amount over a long period of time (such as 100,000 units a day for several months) can cause symptoms of illness, so be careful not to take too much. After you have taken up to 35,000 units for a few months, or when the symptoms of a deficiency disappear, it might be best to limit your vitamin A supplement to about 20,000 units a day. A two-ounce serving of cooked beef liver supplies more than 30,000 units of vitamin A! So you're not talking about a large amount of vitamin A when you talk about 20,000 units.

The carotene in yellow and green vegetables is not toxic. Although carotene can be converted into vitamin A by your body, an excessive amount of carotene (from drinking carrot juice, for example) may turn your skin orange or yellow, but no other ill effects will occur.

*Note:* If you suffer from chronic diarrhea, colitis, gall bladder trouble, or cirrhosis of the liver, or if you have had pancreatic or intestinal surgery, ask your doctor about a possible vitamin A deficiency resulting from your inability to absorb or store fat-soluble vitamins. (If you are a diabetic, your body may not be able to convert carotene into vitamin A.)

Remember that using mineral oil as a laxative will result in elimination of vitamin A through your bowels. When you need a laxative, eat large portions of raw fruits and vegetables which are rich in fiber and vitamin A.

### Vitamin B Complex for Strong, Healthy Nerves

Unlike fat-soluble vitamin A, the B vitamins are water soluble and cannot be stored in your body. An excess of B vitamins is simply eliminated by your kidneys, so you don't have to worry about any toxic effects resulting from taking B vitamins. There are some precautions to be observed, however. Since there are several B vitamins that work together, an excess of one B vitamin might create a deficiency in another B vitamin. Dosing with vitamin $B_6$, for example, increases your body's need for riboflavin; while dosing with riboflavin might produce a $B_6$ deficiency. So it's rarely a good idea to take only one B vitamin unless you have a specific deficiency. Besides, when there is a deficiency in one B vitamin there is likely to be a deficiency in other B vitamins. For this reason, when you feel that you need one of the B vitamins, you should take them all together in a *B-complex* formula.

Remember that since B vitamins are water soluble, you tend to lose them when you have kidney trouble or when you take diuretics.

### *B Vitamins for the Tired Housewife*

If you feel nervous, tired, and exhausted, a high-potency vitamin B-complex supplement might give you a lift. All of the B vitamins play a part in the metabolism of carbohydrate for production of energy. Since vitamin C is also helpful in withstanding nervous stress, vitamin B complex is often combined with vitamin C in what is called "stress formula." You can get it in any drug store or health food store without a prescription.

*Note*: When your kidneys are forced to eliminate excess B vitamins, your urine may change color and odor. This is nothing to be alarmed about, however, if there are no other symptoms.

### *Vitamin $B_1$—the Vigor Vitamin*

A severe deficiency of vitamin $B_1$ (thiamine) results in degeneration of the nervous system (beriberi), a rare disease that must be diagnosed and treated by a physician. The early symptoms of a thiamine deficiency, however, such as nervous exhaustion, fatigue, neuritis, depression, irritability, poor memory, loss of appetite, insomnia, and constipation, can often be eliminated by taking thiamine for a few weeks.

The recommended daily allowance of thiamine is about 1.5 milligrams. Up to 30 milligrams a day, in divided oral doses, are often recommended for treatment purposes. (You can reduce the dosage when you detect the strong odor of thiamine in your urine.)

The best food sources of thiamine are brewer's yeast, whole-grain products, meats (especially pork and liver), peas, beans, and soybeans.

*Note:* Excessive use of sugar, refined carbohydrates, or alcohol can result in a thiamine deficiency. *Natural* carbohydrates contain the thiamine your body needs to metabolize carbohydrate. But refined carbohydrates such as sugar *steal* thiamine and other B vitamins from your body during the metabolic process. So be sure to stick to *natural* foods, as you were instructed to do in chapters 2 and 3.

### Vitamin B₂—the Longevity Vitamin

As in the case of all the B vitamins, you need adequate amounts of vitamin B₂ (riboflavin) to stay healthy and to feel well. Cracks at the corners of the mouth, soreness and redness of the tongue, and a greasy, scaly, red skin around the ears, eyes, and the vaginal opening are the most distinctive symptoms of a riboflavin deficiency. *A prolonged deficiency can result in premature aging and a shortened life.*

You must have at least 1.7 milligrams of riboflavin each day to *prevent* development of deficiency symptoms. Doctors use up to 30 milligrams a day in the *treatment* of a deficiency.

The best sources of riboflavin are milk, cheese, liver, meat, eggs, and brewer's yeast.

*Note:* In addition to being water soluble, riboflavin is destroyed by light. Be sure to observe the cooking procedures recommended in chapter 3.

### Vitamin B₃—the Anti-Pellagra Vitamin

If you're a "corn-fed beauty" and corn is still a major part of your diet, you might tend to be deficient in vitamin B₃, also called niacin or nicotinic acid. In addition to withholding its niacin, corn is deficient in tryptophane, an amino acid that can be converted to niacin by your body.

The early symptoms of a niacin deficiency are loss of appetite, loss of weight, and general weakness. When the deficiency becomes more advanced, the tongue becomes fiery red, the mucous membranes of the mouth and the digestive tract become inflamed, resulting in diarrhea and vomiting. The skin on the hands and feet and around the neck often appears diseased. Nervous and mental symptoms may also appear. Doctors look for three basic symptoms in pellagra: dementia (mental illness), diarrhea, and dermatitis (skin disease).

Fifteen to 20 milligrams of niacin supplied by natural foods would prevent the development of symptoms of pellagra. Once the disease does develop, it is usually treated with 300 to 1,000 milligrams of niacinamide daily in divided oral doses. A large dose of niacin may produce uncomfortable flushing, burning, or itching, but such reactions do not occur with niacinamide, a special form of niacin.

The best food sources of niacin are brewer's yeast, meat, fish, peas, beans, milk, and eggs.

### Vitamin B₆—the Metabolic Vitamin

If you take birth control pills, you might tend to be deficient in vitamin $B_6$ (pyridoxine). In fact, doctors have observed that contraceptive pills make some women depressed and irritable because the pills create a deficiency in vitamins $B_2$, $B_6$, $B_{12}$, C, and folic acid. One researcher has noted that women who take vitamin and mineral supplements along with their birth control pills have 50 percent fewer cases of dry hair and "easily pluckable" hair and 33 percent fewer cases of dry, scaly skin and swollen or bleeding gums than women who take only the pill.

A deficiency in pyridoxine, which is usually the result of interference with absorption of the vitamin, can cause some of the same symptoms seen in other B-vitamin deficiencies, without any characteristic symptoms. So when any of the symptoms of a vitamin B deficiency appear, pyridoxine should be included in a B-complex formula. You need only about two milligrams daily to prevent symptoms of a deficiency, but you may need from 25 to 100 milligrams a day to correct a deficiency. Most high-potency B-complex supplements contain adequate amounts of the major B vitamins.

The best food sources of pyridoxine are brewer's yeast, liver, organ meats, whole-grain cereals, fish, legumes, seeds, and wheat germ.

### Vitamin B₁₂—the Blood Vitamin

Although many of the B vitamins can be found in peas, beans, potatoes, green leafy vegetables, seeds, whole grains, and other foods, *vitamin $B_{12}$ is found almost exclusively in foods of animal origin.* Liver, meats, eggs, milk, and milk products are the principal sources of vitamin $B_{12}$.

When there is not adequate vitamin $B_{12}$ in the diet, a serious form of pernicious anemia might develop. This is why vegetarians are always advised to include dairy products or eggs in their diet.

Actually, only a small amount of vitamin $B_{12}$ is needed for good health. The recommended daily allowance, for example, is only about six micrograms. (Most vitamins are measured in milligrams. A microgram is one-thousandth of a milligram. A milligram is one-thousandth of a gram. A gram is approximately one-thirtieth of an ounce.)

Pernicious anemia that occurs as a result of a *dietary* deficiency in vitamin $B_{12}$ is rare. Most of the time, pernicious anemia occurs as a result of an inability of the stomach to absorb $B_{12}$. This means that the disease must be treated by a physician.

*Warning*: If you develop any of the symptoms of anemia, such as weakness, shortness of breath, rapid heart rate, a sore tongue, or tingling in your hands and feet, have your doctor examine your blood before you try to treat yourself by taking supplements.

### Folic Acid—the Anti-Anemia Vitamin

Folic acid helps prevent anemia. It can also relieve the symptoms of pernicious anemia without *curing* the disease, and this can cause trouble for vegetarians suffering from anemia. Since the principal sources of folic acid are green leafy vegetables and fruits, a strict vegetarian who does not include any animal products in her diet might not experience any of the symptoms of pernicious anemia until the disease is so far advanced that it damages the nervous system.

*Remember*: In addition to being deficient in vitamin $B_{12}$, a strictly vegetarian diet contains enough folic acid to *conceal* anemia caused by a $B_{12}$ deficiency. So, if you don't eat meat, don't be a vegetarian; be a lacto-ovo-vegetarian and include milk or milk products and eggs in your diet.

Because folic acid can mask the symptoms of pernicious anemia, it cannot be purchased in significant amounts without a physician's prescription. Make sure that you and your family get an adequate amount of this vitamin from green leafy vegetables. Other sources are liver, fruits, and brewer's yeast. Folic acid is especially important in preventing anemia during pregnancy.

*Note*: Anemia due to folic acid deficiency is frequently found amoung women who use oral contraceptives. This and other dangers of "the pill" should result in renewed interest in the diaphragm as a method of contraception that can be used without complications.


### The Other B Vitamins

If you eat natural foods that supply the major B vitamins, you'll probably get adequate amounts of the lesser-known B vitamins. Choline, inositol, and pantothenic acid, for example, have important functions in the body, but they may not always be found in B-complex supplements. So you might want to supplement your diet with brewer's yeast and wheat germ for vitamin B insurance. Your body uses choline and inositol, along with pyridoxine, to manufacture lecithin, which helps prevent a buildup of hard fat and cholesterol in your arteries. Soybean lecithin is often used as a supplement to combat hardened arteries and to reduce blood cholesterol.

Pantothenic acid is also useful in preventing a buildup of blood fat and cholesterol, and it is believed to be useful in the treatment of arthritis. In fact, pantothenic acid and pyridoxine are often prescribed in the treatment of arthritis, since both are involved in the body's metabolic processes.

The recommended daily allowance for pantothenic acid is believed to be about 10 milligrams. At least 50 milligrams a day are used in correcting suspected deficiencies.


### Vitamin C—Every Woman's Beauty Vitamin

Because vitamin C (ascorbic acid) is so important in building healthy tissue, it is often called the beauty vitamin. When there is not adequate vitamin C in the diet, tissue cells literally become unglued and fall apart. Tiny blood vessels break, the gums bleed, and teeth loosen. Resistance to infection is lowered and wounds heal slowly. *If you bruise easily, you may be showing early signs of a vitamin C deficiency.*

Since vitamin C is essential in the formation of collagen, a form of connective tissue in the body, you must have more than adequate amounts of vitamin C to keep your skin and your tissues tight and elastic and to prevent premature aging.

Citrus fruits are the best and the most readily available source of vitamin C. Tomatoes, fresh potatoes, cabbage, and green peppers are also good sources.

## Every Woman Needs Extra Vitamin C

Since vitamin C is easily lost in cooking procedures, it's best to depend upon *raw* fruits and vegetables for this important vitamin. You must have at least 60 milligrams a day to prevent symptoms of a deficiency (100 milligrams a day during pregnancy), but you may need considerably more than that for radiant health and beauty.*

Because of the role that vitamin C plays in the prevention of colds and other infections, and its usefulness in lowering blood cholesterol, the authors of this book recommend that every woman take a natural vitamin supplement that supplies a few hundred milligrams of vitamin C daily (along with a balanced diet). During illness, during the cold season, or when fresh fruits aren't available, it might be a good idea to take about 1,000 milligrams a day in divided doses. Since vitamin C is a water-soluble vitamin, any excess will simply be eliminated by the kidneys. Once a saturation level has been reached, as indicated by elimination of vitamin C by the kidneys, an habitual intake of 80 to 100 milligrams of vitamin C daily will probably maintain saturation under normal conditions.

Taking vitamin C in small, divided doses, rather than in one large dose, will help maintain saturation and reduce urinary loss of the vitamin.

*Note*: Whenever vitamin C is excreted in the urine, it may be mistaken for sugar in a urinalysis. So be sure to discontinue use of vitamin C for a couple of days before a scheduled urine test.

## Vitamin D—the Sunshine Vitamin

One of the most important functions of vitamin D is to aid absorption of the calcium and phosphorus you need for strong bones. A deficiency in vitamin D results in osteomalacia, or soft bones. The best food sources of vitamin D are fish liver oil, butter, egg yolk, and liver. Sunlight forms vitamin D on your skin. Whenever you go on a low-fat, low-cholesterol diet, try to expose your skin to sunlight occasionally. (Remember, however, that too much sun ages the skin!) Use skimmed milk that has been enriched with vitamin D. Snack on sunflower seeds for a little extra D. When you take a calcium supplement to strengthen your bones, make sure that it also contains vitamin D and phosphorus.

---

*The Minimum Daily Requirement (MDR) for vitamin C in preventing symptoms of deficiency is usually given as 30 milligrams. The Recommended Daily Allowance (RDA), which may range from 45 to 75 milligrams, is the amount of vitamin C believed needed to maintain good health in a healthy person. No one really knows, however, how much vitamin C is needed for the best of health. Every individual's needs are different.

The recommended daily allowance of vitamin D for healthy adults is 400 U.S.P. units. When you need vitamin D, chances are you also need calcium. So pick a supplement, such as vitamin D enriched bone meal, that supplies about 1,000 milligrams of calcium daily.

*Note:* Since vitamin D is a fat-soluble vitamin, it can be stored in your body. As in the case of vitamin A, you should not take large doses over a long period of time. Too much vitamin D can be toxic, and it can result in absorption of too much calcium (which may accumulate in tissues, blood vessels, and organs).

Ask your doctor about taking more than 1,600 units of vitamin D a day. It usually takes 100,000 units a day for several months to produce toxic effects. But unless your doctor is treating you for a specific disease, it's not likely that you could benefit from more than a couple thousand units a day. Make sure that you get adequate vitamin D during pregnancy and while you are breast feeding your baby.

### Vitamin E—the Anti-Aging Vitamin

Vitamin E used to be known as the fertility vitamin, but it is now best known for its value in improving circulation and protecting the heart. Vitamin E is also an antioxidant; that is, it protects tissue cells and essential fatty acids from the destructive effects of oxygen. Since premature aging has been attributed largely to oxidation, many nutritionists now recommend vitamin E for combating aging and preserving youthfulness. In addition to protecting tissue cells from the aging effects of oxygen, vitamin E *conserves* oxygen in your body, thus relieving the workload on your heart and lungs.

Doctors estimate that you need only about 30 units of vitamin E daily if you are healthy. Surveys, however, indicate that the average American gets less than one-third of the recommended daily allowance of vitamin E. One reason for this, of course, is that few people eat adequate amounts of whole-grain products. Most of the foods in the average diet are processed and refined.

Sprinkle a little wheat germ on whole-grain cereals. Eat a slice of whole-grain bread with each meal. Leafy vegetables and egg yolk supply vitamin E. Vegetable oils also contain vitamin E, but unless the oils are of the cold-pressed variety (as supplied by health food stores) they may create a need for more vitamin E than they supply. (The more fatty acids you have in your diet, the more vitamin E you need to prevent oxidation of the fatty acids. See chapter 5 for additional explanation.) Limit your use of vegetable oil to a few tablespoons daily on a raw salad.

If you want some vitamin E insurance, take about 200 units daily in divided doses. Use a *natural* vitamin E complex, with *mixed* tocopherols.


### Calcium—the Bone Mineral

Your body contains more calcium than any other mineral. You need calcium for strong bones and tight teeth, especially during pregnancy and lactation. If you have gone through your menopause, you may need additional calcium to prevent osteoporosis caused by loss of calcium from your bones. The "dowager's hump," for example, occurs when a calcium deficiency allows vertebrae to soften until they actually collapse.

The recommended daily allowance for calcium is about 1,000 milligrams (one gram). You may need up to 1,500 milligrams daily during pregnancy or if your bones have been softened by osteoporosis. Remember, however, that you must also have adequate vitamin D and phosphorus to utilize calcium. Bone meal tablets (see chapter 5) contain all the minerals you need to build strong bones. Every woman should probably take bone meal tablets after menopause.

*Milk and milk products are the best food sources of calcium.* Green leafy vegetables also supply calcium, but spinach, beet greens, and sorrel contain oxalic acid that prevents utilization of calcium. Try to depend upon milk products for your recommended daily allowance of calcium and then take a calcium supplement when you feel you need additional calcium.

*Note:* The hydrochloric acid in your stomach aids absorption of calcium. Most people tend to be deficient in stomach acid after middle age, however. If your doctor tells you that your bones have softened in spite of a calcium-rich diet, you may have to take a hydrochloric acid supplement along with your meals. Ask your health food store or your druggist for betaine hydrochloride tablets. Discontinue use of the tablets if they seem to cause digestive discomfort.


### Iron—the Blood Mineral

Iron deficiency anemia is fairly common among women who menstruate heavily. The reason for this, of course, is that loss of blood each month results in loss of more iron than the diet supplies. Pregnancy may also create a need for additional iron.

Ordinarily, a diet that supplies 18 milligrams of iron each day would be adequate in maintaining good health. When a deficiency develops, however, doctors may prescribe 300 milligrams of ferrous sulfate or ferrous gluconate three times a day. Since only a small amount of this iron can be absorbed, the treatment is continued for at least two months after the hemoglobin (iron) reaches a normal level. (A female is considered anemic if the iron content of her blood is less than 12 grams per 100 milliliters of blood. Ideally, the hemoglobin level should be about 14 grams.)

Since an excessive amount of iron in the blood can have toxic effects, it's not a good idea to take large doses of iron over a long period of time when there is not an iron deficiency. For this reason, it's always best to have a physician test your blood before taking the amount of iron required to correct an iron-deficiency anemia. There are many different kinds of anemia, and some of them cannot be corrected by taking iron.

You cannot get too much iron from iron-rich natural foods. So try to get all the iron you need from the foods you eat. *Liver is the best source of iron.* Many other foods, such as dried fruits, beans, and leafy vegetables also supply iron. Remember that you need protein as well as iron to form iron-carrying hemoglobin. You also need a variety of other nutrients supplied by a *balanced diet*.

*Note*: If you suffer from weakness, fatigue, and headache, ask your doctor for a complete blood count (CBC). This test will uncover possible anemia.

### Iodine—the Mineral That Prevents Goiter

You need only a tiny amount of iodine for good health. When there is not adequate iodine in your diet, your thyroid gland enlarges, resulting in a simple goiter or enlargement on the front of your neck. Goiter is more common among females than among males, and it usually occurs during puberty, pregnancy, or menopause.

In a few areas of the world where iodine deficiency is the rule rather than the exception, a goiter on the neck of a female is thought of as a mark of beauty. In this country, however, a goiter is recognized as a disease and a deformity. Don't let a simple iodine deficiency spoil your physical beauty!

Once a goiter develops, treatment should be supervised by a physician. Iodine in the form of a medicine can be harmful, since an overdose can result in nervousness and other symptoms of hyperthyroidism.

The best way to get your iodine is to eat seafood, use iodized salt, and take kelp supplements. This way you'll *prevent* development of a goiter and you won't get too much iodine.

## Phosphorus Is Not Often Deficient

Phosphorus is a part of every cell in your body, but its most important function is to combine with calcium to strengthen bones and teeth. Since phosphorus is widely distributed in animal and plant products, it's not likely that you'll ever be deficient in phosphorus if you have a balanced diet. Too much phosphorus supplied by an unbalanced diet can result in urinary loss of calcium. Dietary phosphorus supplied by a high-protein meat diet, for example, without adequate calcium, can literally drain calcium from your body.

Probably the only time you might need to take a phosphorus supplement is when you take a calcium supplement to speed rebuilding of soft bones. The recommended daily allowance for phosphorus is about the same as that for calcium: 1,000 milligrams (one gram). The ratio of calcium to phosphorus in bone meal is about two to one. Your diet will supply additional phosphorus.

Remember that *prevention* is the best approach to good health. If you want to maintain good health, eat a variety of natural foods and let nature balance the essential nutrients needed by your body.

## SUMMARY

1. Every woman should depend first upon a balanced diet of natural foods for the essential nutrients and then take supplements when the need arises.

2. Vitamin A is essential in maintaining a beautiful skin and a high resistance to infection.

3. When you need vitamin B for your nerves, always take vitamin B complex so that you won't create an imbalance in the B vitamins.

4. Anemia can result from a deficiency in vitamin $B_{12}$, iron, or folic acid, as well as from a number of other causes. Always find out what type of anemia you have before attempting self-treatment.

5. Vitamin C keeps your tissues healthy and elastic and helps prevent infection.

6. When you take calcium to harden your bones after menopause, remember that you also need vitamin D and phosphorus to utilize the calcium.

7. Vitamin E improves circulation and helps delay the aging process by preventing oxidation of tissue cells and essential fatty acids.

8. Iodine supplied by seafood, iodized salt, and kelp products helps protect against development of a goiter.

9. Excessive amounts of vitamins A and D in supplement form can have harmful effects but are harmless in natural foods.

10. If you have a specific intestinal or digestive disorder, ask your doctor if there is likely to be interference with absorption of certain vitamins or minerals.

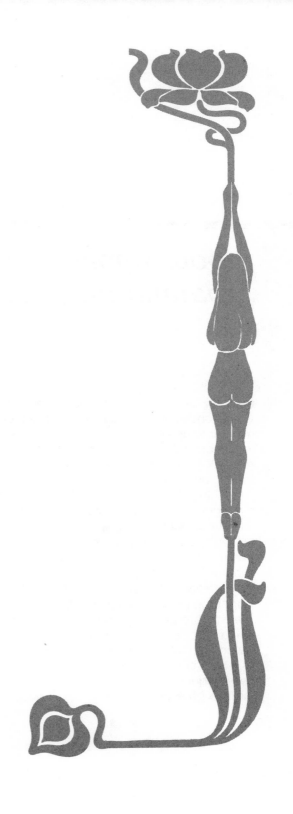

# food supplements for maintaining good health

In chapter 2 you learned that "natural foods" are simply fresh foods that can be purchased in any grocery store. In chapter 4, you were told which foods contained the essential nutrients and how to take vitamin and mineral supplements. In this chapter you'll learn about certain *concentrated* natural food substances that are so potent in their vitamin and mineral content that they can serve as *supplements* in building or maintaining good health.

Actually, there are a couple of good reasons why you should depend first upon natural food substances for your vitamins and minerals rather than upon tablets or capsules that supply isolated nutrients. For one thing, there are many *undiscovered nutrients* in a natural food substance. Some of these nutrients help your body absorb and utilize vitamins and minerals. For example, we know that calcium cannot be utilized in the construction of bones without vitamin D. There are several B vitamins that work together to support the function of one B vitamin. The oil-soluble vitamins are best absorbed in the natural oils in which they are normally found. Vitamin C may be more effective when it is accompanied by bioflavonoids, rutin, and other naturally associated nutrients.

Your body's utilization of nutrients is a complicated, overlapping process, requiring a great variety of known and unknown nutrients to maintain the balance needed for good health. For this reason, it might be a

90

# Chapter 5

good idea to use natural food substances, whenever possible, to correct a deficiency so that you'll be assured of getting all the nutrients you need. Bone meal, for example, supplies calcium, phosphorus, vitamin D, magnesium, zinc, and other minerals you need for strong bones and good teeth. Brewer's yeast contains *all* the B vitamins you need for healthy nerves. Desiccated liver supplies vitamin $B_{12}$ as well as iron for building rich, red blood.

### Lynda Day George—Versatile Femininity

When beautiful, feminine Lynda Day George is not acting before movie or television cameras or on the stage, she might be found doing electrical, plumbing, or carpentry work in her home! Or she might be working on her health-and-beauty book. With a husband, two children, a busy acting schedule, a book project, and a variety of constructive hobbies, Lynda George obviously finds time to practice the health and beauty secrets she plans to reveal in the book she is writing. Most women would be interested in knowing, for example, that she shampoos her hair *every morning* when she is working. And she sometimes uses mayonnaise

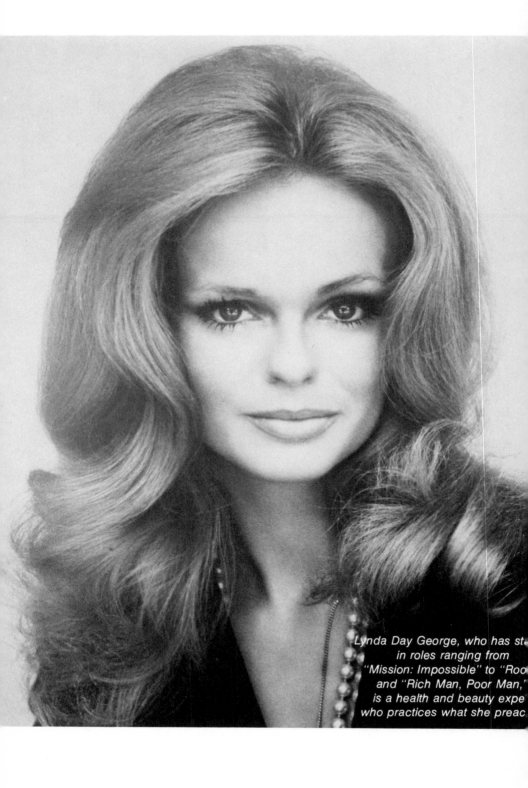

Lynda Day George, who has st[ar]
in roles ranging from
"Mission: Impossible" to "Roo[ts]
and "Rich Man, Poor Man,"
is a health and beauty expe[rt]
who practices what she preac[hes]

on her hair to restore lost oil. It may surprise most women to learn that this glamorous star does not use makeup on her skin when she is not performing before cameras or an audience.

"A good, balanced diet that avoids sugars, additives, and fats is a woman's best bet for good skin," she advises, "provided, of course, you keep your skin *clean*."

Good nutrition plays an important role in Lynda George's health and beauty program. And with gourmet cooking as a hobby, she often prepares unusual dishes that are highly nutritious. For added health insurance, she supplements her diet with selected nutrients. "Each morning," she says, "I have a protein drink made with fruit, cream, and powdered protein. This holds me until around 3 P.M. when I eat and take my regular vitamin supplements containing A, B complex, C, E, and lecithin. In the evening I take calcium, iron, and other minerals."

Lynda Day George favors a high-protein, low-carbohydrate diet, but she feels that "most of us in this country 'over-protein' ourselves into old age."

Although the health and beauty secrets of beautiful, glamorous women often differ when it comes to such personal habits as hair and skin care, practically all of them use dietary supplements. You should, too, if you want the nutritional insurance you need for lasting health and beauty. But you should first acquire the knowledge you need to select the nutrients you need most. So be sure to continue your study of nutrition, even after reading this book.

## Basic Food Supplements for Every Woman

There are many tasty, wholesome food substances that you can use in your health and beautification program. Remember that good nutrition is an important factor in physical beauty. Without healthy skin, elastic tissues, shiny hair, and youthful verve, all of the cosmetics in the world cannot give you what you need to be truly beautiful.

Once you have acquired a good basic knowledge of how to improve your health with foods and natural food substances, you'll benefit more from the specific measures recommended in the final chapters of this book. In the meantime, remember that you can literally *eat* your way to good health! *Every woman can safely and effectively use the 10 food substances described in this chapter.*

### Brewer's Yeast for Super Energy

Brewer's yeast is a very potent natural food substance. In addition to containing all the known B vitamins, it supplies some very important trace minerals such as selenium and chromium. *Selenium*, like vitamin E, is an antioxidant that delays the aging process by protecting tissue cells and essential fatty acids from damage by oxygen. *Chromium* aids sugar metabolism and helps protect against the development of diabetes and hypoglycemia. Some nutritionists believe that the chromium content of yeast will help prevent overweight. Brewer's yeast is also the richest available source of the nucleic acids DNA and RNA, which are believed to be helpful in delaying the aging process.

### *How to Take Yeast*

Three or four tablespoons of brewer's yeast powder each day can do wonders in waking up tired nerves, controlling your blood sugar, and protecting your health. Brewer's yeast is more potent in powder form than in tablet form. It takes about 15 tablets, for example, to equal two tablespoons of powder. Persons who do not like the taste of yeast, however, will prefer to take the tablets.

There are many ways to take yeast powder. You can mix it in milk, soup, juices, peanut butter, homemade bread, meat loaf, or any food you like. The stronger the flavor of the food, the more yeast you can add. If you use a small amount of powder several times a day, however, you can get your quota of yeast without being overwhelmed by the taste. Once you have become accustomed to taking yeast, you'll begin to enjoy the flavor.

*Caution*: Since brewer's yeast is very rich in phosphorus, it might be a good idea to take a calcium lactate tablet along with yeast to make sure there is no urinary loss of calcium, especially when you are pregnant or breast feeding.

One of the best ways to take yeast powder is to make a *Sunshine Cocktail*. The calcium in the milk will help balance the phosphorus

---

### sunshine cocktail

Combine one quart milk with one-half cup dried milk, one-half cup brewer's yeast powder, and a small can of frozen, concentrated orange juice.

Mix in a blender and keep in a refrigerator for use throughout the day or when you feel you need a lift.

supplied by the yeast. If you are pregnant, however, take a calcium lactate tablet with each glass of Sunshine Cocktail.

### Brewer's Yeast vs. Baker's Yeast

When you use yeast as a food supplement, be sure to use *brewer's* yeast and not baker's yeast. The type of yeast used in baking contains *live* yeast plants that will steal nutrients from your intestinal tract. Of course, the heat used in baking kills the live plants so that they can be easily digested.

There are other types of food yeast or nutritional yeast that are grown in a different manner from brewer's yeast. All of these yeasts are highly nutritious. But since they may not measure up to brewer's yeast in chromium content, always select *brewer's* yeast whenever you have a choice.

*Note:* If brewer's yeast taken with meals seems to give you gas, try taking your yeast in tablet form between meals.

### Wheat Germ for "Staying Power"

Wheat germ follows close behind brewer's yeast as a source of protein and B vitamins. It's the *vitamin E* in wheat germ, however, that gives it special appeal. And wheat germ is *delicious!* You can eat it as a cereal or add it to other cereals. It can be added to homemade bread, cookies, or meat loaf. It can be sprinkled over anything from fried pork chops to ice cream. Some health food cooks use wheat germ instead of bread crumbs in cooking.

Many athletes use wheat germ and wheat germ oil to increase their endurance or "staying power." Some researchers believe that there is something in wheat germ oil (other than vitamin E) that increases physical endurance. If you're a busy housewife with a large family, you need as much endurance as any athlete. So why not include wheat germ in your diet? Vitamin E supplied by wheat germ oil might be useful in correcting problems in your reproductive organs and in easing the strain of menopause. There's a possibility that wheat germ oil might even add a little "staying power" to your sex life. (Feed wheat germ oil to your man when he seems to be lagging!)

*Note:* Since wheat germ and wheat germ oil will spoil or turn rancid quite easily, keep them in closed containers in your refrigerator. Use them daily so that you don't have to keep them too long. Don't use them if they become rancid.

You can purchase *raw* wheat germ in health food stores, but the toasted variety, available in any grocery store, is tastier and easier to use.

*Caution*: If you eat large amounts of wheat germ, be sure to take a calcium supplement such as calcium lactate to balance the phosphorus supplied by the wheat germ. (Bone meal is a good natural source of calcium.)

### Bone Meal for Strong Hips and a Straight Spine

You know from reading chapter 4 that bone meal supplies balanced amounts of all the minerals you need to keep your bones strong. Taking two 10-grain tablets of bone meal with each meal, for example, will provide slightly more than your recommended daily allowance of calcium. (Make sure that the bone meal you use has been enriched with vitamin D.)

The older you become, the more important it is to take a bone meal supplement. Most women tend to lose calcium from their bones after menopause. This is most often the result of a decline in the body's production of estrogen hormones. But it can also result from a simple dietary deficiency and from physical inactivity. *Be sure to get plenty of exercise* (see chapter 9). Your bones will absorb only the amount of calcium they need to withstand the amount of stress you place upon them. If you never exercise, your bones may get so weak that they'll fracture quite easily.

Some doctors routinely recommend use of estrogen to strengthen soft bones after menopause. Since estrogen might trigger the growth of a latent malignancy, however, you should make sure that you are getting adequate dietary calcium and sufficient exercise before considering use of hormones to harden your bones.

When your upper back begins to show evidence of slumping into a hump, see an orthopedic specialist for an examination and then get on a high-protein diet supplemented with bone meal or a capsule containing calcium, phosphorus, and vitamin D. (Chapter 11 describes a special exercise that you can use to reverse a slump in your back.)

#### What One Woman Did About a Slumped Spine

The case of Claire C. is a good example of how the development of a slumped spine or a "dowager's hump" can be halted after menopause. Claire had been a bank teller for 38 years! At the age of 60, she had only a few more years to go before retirement. Since the age of 58, however, she had complained of an increasing amount of pain and fatigue in her upper back, and her spine was obviously slumping. When her work, which required standing behind a bank counter, became unbearable, she made an appointment with her family doctor, who ordered an x-ray examination. "You have osteoporosis," he told her, "which means that you have a calcium deficiency in your bones. Your vertebrae are getting soft."

"But I drink plenty of milk," she insisted. "How come I'm deficient in calcium?"

Good question!

Since Claire was probably not absorbing her calcium, she was instructed to take a betaine hydrochloride supplement along with bone meal and vitamin D. Miraculously, her bones began to harden and further compression of her vertebrae was halted.

Claire was lucky. In a few more years, the uncorrected deficiency would have resulted in a painful, disfiguring "dowager's hump" that would have been a permanent deformity.

### How to Take Bone Meal

Bone meal is probably more easily absorbed in powder form than in tablet form. But since the odor and taste of bone meal leave much to be desired, most people prefer to take the tablets. Bone meal powder can, however, be used in cooking. You can mix the powder into bread dough or meat loaf, for example, or you can mix it with peanut butter or homemade confections. As in the case of most natural food supplements, you cannot take too much bone meal. There are no side effects to worry about, so try to include bone meal in your diet whether you think you need it or not.

Betaine hydrochloride, which aids absorption of calcium (when accompanied by vitamin D), can be purchased in any health food store (see chapter 4).

### Prevent a Broken Hip with Bone Meal

Like the dowager's hump, hip fracture is common among elderly women and is most often the result of a calcium deficiency. In some cases, when the deficiency is severe, a hip will fracture spontaneously while *walking*, causing a fall that is falsely believed to be the *cause* of the fracture. If your bones are strong and your diet contains adequate calcium, you're not likely to break a bone, no matter how old you might be. Bone meal might be the answer.

### Desiccated Liver Combats Fatigue

If you suffer from "tired blood" (a catchy advertising description of simple anemia), you may find a miraculous cure in desiccated or dried liver. In tablet form for easy consumption, dried liver supplies B vitamins and protein along with the iron and $B_{12}$ your body needs to build iron-rich blood cells.

You should, of course, eat *fresh* liver at least once a week whenever possible. But if you want extra blood-building nutrients to protect your health (especially during menstrual periods) without having to eat heavily, take a few desiccated liver tablets along with your other nutritional supplements.

*Brewer's yeast and desiccated liver taken together offer the best possible source of the iron and B vitamins you need for youthful verve.* Liver also contains some unknown substance known as the "anti-fatigue factor," and it contains other factors not found in yeast. Taken together, liver and yeast are truly wonder foods.

### How to Add Skimmed Milk Powder to Your Diet

If you tolerate milk very well and you need a high-protein drink to supplement your diet, you may simply mix a few tablespoons of powdered skimmed milk into a glass of skimmed milk. Adding one cup of skimmed milk powder to one quart (four cups) of skimmed milk will provide about 65 grams of protein, your recommended daily allowance. You may enrich the milk with additional powder if you like. (Each cup of skimmed milk powder contains about 29 grams of protein.)

Skimmed milk powder can be used in many ways when cooking. It can be added to any food recipe in which milk is an ingredient. Remember that if you cannot tolerate the lactose in milk, you convert the lactose to lactic acid by *fermenting* your milk. You learned in chapter 3 how to make skimmed milk yogurt. For a *high-protein yogurt*, add a little powdered skimmed milk to skimmed milk before adding the lactobacillus.

### Lecithin and Vegetable Oil Help Blood Circulate

The B vitamins (choline and inositol) and fatty acids supplied by lecithin and vegetable oil are essential for healthy skin. They are also essential for good blood circulation and a long life. Without the soft fat supplied by essential fatty acids, the hard fat and cholesterol in your blood would harden and clog your arteries. The danger of this is greater after menopause.

You can help protect your arteries by taking a little lecithin each day or by adding a few tablespoons of cold-pressed vegetable oil to a raw salad. Safflower oil is the richest source of linoleic acid, the most important essential fatty acid. Sunflower seeds are also a good source of linoleic acid. Mayonnaise made of vegetable oil is rich in essential fatty acids. If you're not overweight, you can use a little mayonnaise occasionally on salads. To make sure that the mayonnaise you use does not contain sugar or artificial additives, however, you should make your own by combining eggs, salad oil, vinegar, and lemon juice.

It goes without saying that you must cut down on animal fat if you want to keep your blood cholesterol down. If there is more hard fat than soft fat in your blood, the hard fat will clump together and clog your arteries.

### Combine Vitamin E with Vegetable Oil

Although vegetable oil contains vitamin E, remember that it might be helpful to take a little vitamin E with vegetable oils. You know from reading chapter 4 that you must have vitamin E to prevent oxidation of the essential fatty acids supplied by oil. Since most vegetable oils, even the cold-pressed variety, have been processed enough to cause some loss of this vitamin, you should not depend upon vegetable oil alone for vitamin E—*with the exception of wheat germ oil.*

If you use more than a few tablespoons of vegetable oil daily (for skin problems or for some other reason), include a vitamin E supplement. Since vitamin E opens blood vessels and helps prevent the formation of blood clots, you can get double protection from combining vegetable oil and vitamin E.

### How to Use Lecithin

Lecithin is usually extracted from soybeans. In granule or powdered form, it can be sprinkled over foods. In liquid form, it can be stirred into beverages or into "health drinks."

If you have a gallstone, lecithin added to your diet might help dissolve the cholesterol forming the stone. It is well known that lecithin manufactured by your body is important in keeping cholesterol emulsified in your gall bladder to *prevent* the formation of stones. (Although the digestive process breaks dietary lecithin down into its component parts, your body can reassemble these parts in forming its own lecithin.)

### Kelp for Iodine and Trace Minerals

If you happen to live around the Great Lakes or the Rocky Mountains, where the soil and water do not contain iodine, you won't be able to depend upon home-grown foods for iodine. You'll have to make sure that you use iodized salt or eat seafood regularly. Or you can use kelp supplements supplied by your local health food store.

Kelp, which is simply dried seaweed, is rich in iodine and other trace minerals. Unlike prescription iodine, you cannot get too much iodine from moderate use of kelp. You can eat dried kelp or you can take it in tablet form. You can sprinkle powdered kelp (instead of salt) over your foods.

### *Kelp and a Low-Sodium Diet*

Kelp contains about one-tenth the amount of sodium found in salt, and 10 times as much iodine as iodized salt. If you're on a low-sodium diet, and you don't eat much seafood, you can get your iodine by using powdered kelp instead of salt. You should try to eat seafood occasionally, however, whether you like it or not. Remember that it's difficult to get enough iodine if you do not eat seafood, use iodized salt, or supplement your diet with kelp products.

### Fish Liver Oil for Sunlight Deficiency

If you are a hard-working woman and you spend most of your time indoors or in an office, you may not be able to depend upon sunlight for your vitamin D. Even if you spend a little time outdoors in the city, streets shaded by tall buildings and smog might deprive you of healthful sun rays. You can make sure that you get adequate vitamin D (and vitamin A) by taking fish liver oil.

Animal fat contains some vitamin D, but it also contains saturated fat, of which you should eat as little as possible. Fish liver oil is *unsaturated* and won't contribute to a buildup of cholesterol and hard fat in your arteries.

One quart of enriched milk contains the recommended daily allowance of vitamin D (400 U.S.P. units), but it's difficult for most of us to drink a quart of milk daily. If you include calcium supplements in your diet, you might be able to use a little extra vitamin D for super health and superior beauty. So why not include a little fish liver oil in your supplement program? When you purchase *natural* vitamin D in capsule form, chances are it will be made of fish liver oil. (You'll taste it when you burp!) Read the label to make sure that you're getting pure fish liver oil.

Remember that you need extra vitamin D to help your body absorb and utilize bone-building calcium during pregnancy and after menopause.

### Rose Hips for Megavitamin C

Citrus fruits are our best and most readily available source of vitamin C, but if you want a really concentrated food substance to enrich your diet

---

**how to make rose hip extract**

Here's a simple way to prepare a rose hip extract for use in beverages:

Place the gathered rose hips in a refrigerator and leave them there until they are chilled. This will destroy the enzymes that might react with the vitamin C during preparation of the extract.

Remove all stems and blossom ends and wash the rose hips under running water for a few seconds.

Boil one and a half cups of water for each cup of rose hips. Add chopped or mashed rose hips (preferably liquified in a blender) to the hot water and let the mixture simmer for 15 minutes in a tightly covered saucepan.

Keep the mixture covered and let it stand for 24 hours in a refrigerator. Then strain the extract and bring it to a boil. After it cools, add two tablespoons lemon juice for each pint of extract. Seal in glass jars and store in a refrigerator.

Add one tablespoon of the extract to each glass of fruit or vegetable juice you drink. You may also add the extract to salads, soups, and other foods.

Be sure to use glass, stainless steel, or enameled utensils when preparing rose hip extract. Contact with iron or copper will destroy vitamin C.

with vitamin C, gather a few rose hips. A rose hip is the pod or nodule that's left over when all the rose petals have fallen away. The hips of wild roses contain 10 to 100 times more vitamin C than fresh orange juice! The best time to gather rose hips is when they are bright red or orange in color.

Every health food store stocks rose hip products for use in a variety of ways. You can even make *rose hip tea* with specially prepared tea bags. And, of course, you can purchase natural vitamin C made of rose hips.

## SUMMARY

1. You can increase your intake of essential vitamins and minerals by adding brewer's yeast, wheat germ, bone meal, desiccated liver, skimmed milk powder, lecithin, vegetable oil, kelp, fish liver oil, and rose hip products to your diet.

2. Concentrated natural food substances that supply essential vitamins and minerals also supply other known and unknown nutrients that are vital for radiant health and beauty.

3. Brewer's yeast and desiccated liver combined supply B vitamins and blood-building nutrients that contribute to youthful verve.

4. Wheat germ is rich in vitamin E as well as in B vitamins and protein. Wheat germ *oil* contains some unknown substance that increases physical endurance.

5. If you use a large amount of brewer's yeast or wheat germ, you should include bone meal or calcium lactate to balance your intake of phosphorus.

6. Taking skimmed milk enriched with skimmed milk powder and bone meal enriched with vitamin D, will help prevent bone softening after menopause.

7. Lecithin and cold-pressed vegetable oil supply B vitamins and essential fatty acids that may help prevent clogged arteries and gallstones.

8. Persons who spend all their time indoors should supplement their diet with fish liver oil for vitamin D.

9. If you do not eat seafood or use iodized salt, you can get the iodine you need from kelp products.

10. Rose hips harvested when the pods of wild roses are bright red are very rich in vitamin C.

# special aids for beautification of hair, skin, and nails

Remember what you learned in chapter 1, that the *real* secret of beauty is *good health*? This is especially true in the case of your hair, skin, and nails. Without nourishment from *inside* your body, your skin would become diseased, your hair would fall out or break off, and your nails would crack or split. According to *Human Nutrition* (U.S. Department of Agriculture): "Changes in the skin and hair are often the first indication of nutritional deficiency."

It is very important that you eat properly to get all the nutrients you need to be healthy inside and beautiful outside, so be sure to put into practice what you have learned from reading the previous chapters of this book. In the meantime, there are some basic procedures and a few tricks that you can use in the care of your hair, skin, and nails to make them naturally beautiful *now*—without the use of expensive cosmetics.

There's an ancient maxim that says, "A fair exterior is a silent recommendation." There's no doubt that the first impression you make on people can be very important in everything you do. The impression you make will be determined largely by the appearance of your hair and your skin.

### The Lesson Carolyn Learned

Carolyn T. learned the hard way that her physical appearance could affect her marriage and her career. When her

# Chapter 6

husband began to get involved with another woman and she failed to get the job promotion she expected, she took a good look at herself in a mirror. What she saw was horrifying. Her hair was so oily that it sagged heavily. Flakes of skin from a scaly scalp dotted the hair strands and showed up conspicuously on the dark collar of her blouse. The color of her makeup contrasted sharply with the pale skin of her face. Even the thickest layer of makeup failed to conceal acne-like eruptions on her chin and her forehead. Enlarged pores in her nose were clogged with dark deposits. Her entire body was marred by blemishes and spotty eruptions that were accentuated by white, soggy skin. Cosmetics were obviously not the answer to her problems.

Use of some of the procedures outlined in this chapter resulted in miraculous changes in Carolyn's physical appearance. Restoration of the natural beauty of her hair and her skin with *simple methods of cleaning and grooming* transformed her from a "painted mannequin" to a beautiful, radiant woman! Needless to say, with an improvement in her physical appearance, Carolyn got her husband back. She even got the promotion she wanted when her employer moved her up to a front desk. "I always thought that I was using my cosmetics improperly," she confessed, "but I guess nothing beats soap and water."

Don't let your natural beauty deteriorate to the point where you must hide behind wigs and makeup. Remember that when your hair and skin are clean and healthy, they are beautiful *without* makeup.

## How to Keep Your Hair Beautiful and Manageable

Your hair is literally your crowning glory. When hair is healthy and *clean*, it's naturally elastic and shiny, and it's always receptive to a caressing touch. Try to select a hair style that permits daily brushing and combing. You should be able to play a game of tennis or go to bed with your man without worrying about mussing your hair. If your hair is properly cut, cleaned, and styled, you can quickly fix it with a few strokes of a brush or a comb.

Unfortunately, it is popular among many women today to tease the hair until it is as fluffy as cotton candy. Then, after a little combing over the surface, the hair is sprayed with a sticky lacquer to hold it in a permanent position. In many cases, the same hairdo will be maintained for several days simply by touching up the hair with additional spray. It's okay to style your hair this way on special occasions for short periods of time. But if you go for days without brushing or combing your hair, or if you do not shampoo your hair often, you may be inviting trouble.

Assuming that you are getting adequate nutrients from a balanced diet, and you have normal, healthy hair, many of the problems you have with your hair may be the result of improper care of your scalp.

### Keep Your Scalp Clean

The scalp is normally the oiliest part of the body. Although a dry scalp is a common complaint, some dermatologists say that there is no such thing. What really happens, they say, is that failure to wash the scalp often enough or thoroughly enough allows oil and dead skin to accumulate on the scalp and form a paste that seals pores and oil glands. The result is that the scalp becomes scaly and itchy and the hair dry and dull. Since many people are under the impression that soap and water will make the scalp dry, it's a common mistake to refrain from washing the scalp when it appears to be scaly. Actually, washing the scalp with soap or a shampoo will remove the pasty scale on the scalp so that fresh oil can once again flow from the oil glands around the hair roots. Brushing the hair will then distribute the oil over the hair shafts to make the hair moist and shiny.

Some women who have a dry scalp because of inadequate washing sometimes add oil to their hair to relieve the dryness. This only aggravates the problem by increasing the buildup of scalp paste until the scalp becomes crusted and inflamed. You should wash your head often to remove accumulated scale on your scalp. You can't do this if you wear the same lacquered hairdo for days at a time. And it's not likely that you'll be inclined to groom your hair every day if you put on a wig every time you go out.

*Note*: If you feel that your scalp and your hair are truly too dry after washing, you can use a shampoo that has been designed for use on dry hair, and, if necessary, you can use a creme rinse after shampooing.

Remember that excessive exposure to sun, salt water, or chlorinated water during the swimming season can temporarily dry out normal hair.

See a dermatologist if a scalp problem of any kind persists in spite of regular cleaning.

### You Rarely Need Special Soaps or Shampoos

The average woman should use a basic soap or shampoo that will remove dirt and oil from the scalp without leaving a coating on the hair. Remember that your hair is actually dead. It cannot absorb protein or change its structure in response to a rinse. (If your hair grows out strong and healthy, it will stay that way, just as it does in a wig made of healthy hair. Any changes in the structure of your hair must take place in the roots where it grows.) When the hair is coated with oil, protein, or some other substance left over from a soap or shampoo, the coated hair tends to collect dirt and more oil, requiring even more washing to remove the ever-thickening and stiffening coating.

If your hair has been damaged by chemicals or is so fine and thin that it's difficult to style after washing, you can use a protein conditioner to fill in cracks and splits and to give your hair body. Make sure, however, that you discontinue the use of damaging dyes and other chemicals so that your hair will have a chance to grow out full and strong.

You can make sure that your hair gets all the protein and other nutrients it needs by eating properly. Concentrate on keeping your scalp clean by washing it at least twice a week with a simple, mild soap or shampoo. If you have an excessively oily scalp, wash it as often as necessary to keep your hair from being too oily. Soap and water won't harm healthy hair, so don't be afraid to wash your head. Daily brushing with a *soft* brush will keep dirt-catching oil and dead skin (dandruff) from accumulating on your scalp. Remember, however, that excessive or overly vigorous brushing can damage or break your hair.

### Soaps, Shampoos, and Hard Water

When you wash your hair with soap and hard water, the alkali in the soap combines with the calcium and other minerals in the water to leave a hard, white film on your hair. You can remove this film with a vinegar or lemon rinse.

Squeeze the juice of one lemon into a basin of water, or add one teaspoon of white vinegar to each glass of water poured into a basin. After you have rinsed your hair with one of these solutions, a fresh-water rinse will wash away the accumulated minerals.

Unless you use a water softener in your home, the water from your faucet is likely to be hard water. So if you don't want to use a vinegar or lemon rinse after you wash your hair, *use a detergent shampoo instead of soap*. A detergent that does not contain soap or alkali will not combine with the calcium and magnesium in hard water. (Practically all shampoos are synthetic detergents and do not contain soap.)

*Warning*: Discontinue use of any detergent shampoo that seems to result in an allergic reaction on your scalp or your hands.

It wouldn't be a good idea to install a water softener in your home just to make it easier to wash your hair with soap. Artificially softened water is rich in harmful sodium and low in essential minerals and does not make healthful drinking water.

*Rain water* is soft water. If you have a rain barrel, you might be able to collect enough rain water to use occasionally in washing your hair with soap.

Dry your hair by wrapping it in a towel to absorb the water by blotting. Use a wide-toothed comb to comb wet hair. If you have damaged or thin hair that tangles badly or is too fluffy to comb after washing or drying, you can use a creme rinse or a conditioner after shampooing or washing with soap.

### Hair Loss Can Be Prevented

Baldness in men is caused primarily by the male hormone testosterone, which means that very little can be done to prevent it. When a woman begins to lose hair, however, the cause can often be corrected or eliminated.

Unfortunately, hair loss is becoming increasingly more common among women. Some hair loss may result from the use of wigs and hair styles that do not permit daily combing and frequent washing. Harsh alkaline chemicals used in dyeing and waving hair can cause hair to break off at the scalp. Hair rolled tightly in curlers or brushed too vigorously may damage hair roots, causing them to stop producing hair.

Don't sleep in rollers! And don't pull your hair back tightly with clamps or rubber bands. Let your hair hang free whenever possible.

## Special Attention for Your Face

The skin on the face is normally just about as oily as the scalp. Large pores around the nose and the cheeks collect this oil, creating difficult cleaning problems. If you have blackheads on your face, you already have a cleaning problem. If you're using creams and pancake makeup on your face, you may be *aggravating* the problem. Anything that interferes with the free flow of oil from the pores of the face will enlarge the pores by forcing them to accumulate oil. This can increase the size of blackheads or lead to the development of acne, so it's very important to eliminate the cause of blackheads rather than attempting to hide them with makeup.

Aniko Farrell, a former "Miss Canada" and "Miss World," has beautiful skin that does not require dressing up with cosmetics. "I really don't do a lot regarding skin care," she explains, "because, thank God, I've never had any problem there. I use only soap and cold water on my face, and I never use creams, as I believe they clog up all my pores."

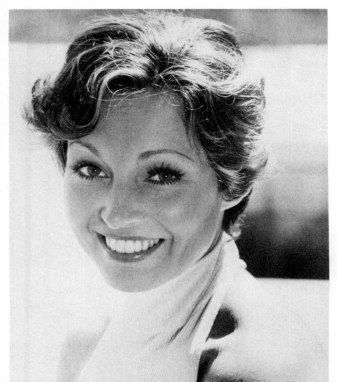

*Aniko Farrell,
a former "Miss Canada"
and "Miss World,"
is married to Peter Palmer,
the movie and Broadway
"Li'l Abner"*

### Soap and Water vs. Cleansing Creams

The best way to clean your face is to use soap and water. *And the oilier your face is, the more washing it needs*. A young woman suffering from acne caused by oily skin may find it necessary to wash her face several times a day with a strongly alkaline soap in order to dissolve the oil accumulating in the pores. It may, in fact, be necessary to wash oily skin until it becomes so dry that it actually *peels*.

You'll have to determine for yourself how much washing your face needs, depending upon how oily it is. Just make sure that you wash your face often enough and thoroughly enough to dissolve the oil in the pores around your nose and your cheeks. Then, if possible, avoid using makeup that interferes with the flow of oil from these pores. If you do apply such makeup occasionally, clean your face thoroughly at the end of the day so that the pores can empty their oil. If you develop the habit of cleaning your face properly while you are still young, you may be able to *prevent* enlargement of facial pores.

There are a few women who are blessed with such small facial pores that they can use cleansing creams for a lifetime without any trouble. Such women are rare, however, and the average woman must make a special effort to keep her pores open and free from clogging. *If you have large pores that seem to accumulate oil and blackheads, you should use soap and water rather than cleansing creams*. Astringents might be helpful in cleaning and tightening large pores.

### How to Empty Clogged Pores

Once the pores of your face have become clogged with hardened oil, it's important to empty those pores to prevent further enlargement. In

---

**formulas for homemade astringents**

Use either a facial mask or liquid astringent with alcohol to dry out oily skin.

*Facial mask:* Mix two tablespoons alcohol with each tablespoon of fuller's earth or clay mask to make a paste. Apply to the skin, let dry, and wash off with warm water. Splash cold water on your face after using the mask.

*Liquid astringent:* Mix four ounces alcohol with four ounces distilled water and one-half teaspoon alum. Dab the solution on the oily areas of your face, particularly around your nose.

some cases simple washing won't do the job. To make sure that you get these pores emptied so that they can be kept clean, follow this procedure:

First wash your face and hands with soap and water to wash away dirt and germs. Then apply hot, moist towels to your face for a few minutes to soften the oil in the clogged pores. Use your fingertips (not your fingernails!) to *gently* press out the hardened oil. Follow this with a hot soap-and-water shower for deep cleansing of the empty pores. Dab on a little alcohol or homemade astringent to guard against infection.

It's always best to clean your pores at night just before retiring so that you won't have to go out in public with a red, splotchy face. Change your pillowcase so that the freshly opened pores won't be exposed to dirt and germs.

Once your pores have been cleaned and opened, keep them clean with a daily soap-and-water *shower.* Don't use creams and pancake makeup. If you care for your face properly, you won't have to clean out your pores more often than a few times a month. Too much pressing of pores as a result of inadequate cleaning may be damaging to the deep tissues of your face, so don't do it too often. But remember that trying to cover up blackheads with makeup on a permanent basis will only breed more blackheads.

*Note:* While it's all right to press an oil plug out of a clogged pore, you should never squeeze a sore or swollen bump. Squeezing an infected pore or oil gland may spread the infection deeper into the tissues and cause a boil or a carbuncle. It is sometimes necessary, however, to open a bump so that it can empty its contents. Use a sterile needle *after* you have cleaned your skin and then dab on a little alcohol. If you suffer from acne, see a dermatologist about opening deep bumps.

### How to Use Beauty Grains

Scrubbing grains, also called "beauty grains," may be helpful in cleaning oily, blemished skin. Soaps containing these grains serve as an abrasive that removes dead skin and rubs away thin skin covering clogged pores and oil glands. Wet oatmeal and cornmeal also make an effective abrasive when rubbed on the skin. Just be careful not to irritate your skin with excessive rubbing, and don't rub around your eyes. A little scrubbing with an abrasive material will leave your skin pink, soft, and glowing. (You can get similar results with a complexion brush or pad.)

### Skin Care Below Your Neck

The skin of your body does not produce as much oil as your face or your scalp and therefore needs less washing. In fact, too much washing with soap may wash away the oils and the acid secretions that protect your skin, leaving it irritated and susceptible to infection.

Use a mild or neutral soap to wash away body oil and dirt. Strongly alkaline soaps should be reserved for acne, dirty hands, and excessively oily skin. The more alkaline the soap, the more cleaning power it has, but also the more irritating it is to the skin. When you do bathe with a strongly alkaline soap, a fresh-water rinse containing a small amount of lemon juice or vinegar will help restore the acid mantle of your skin. (Normal skin quickly restores its acid mantle after washing and won't be harmed by mildly alkaline soap.)

The amount of washing required by your body will depend largely upon the amount of oil being secreted by your skin. If your skin is *normal or oily*, a daily complete body bath with soap and water, with special attention to your face, will be absolutely essential for cleanliness. And the oilier your skin is, the more soap and water you should use. If your skin is *dry*, however, you may have to limit use of soap to your face, armpits, genitals, and feet and then bathe the rest of your body in plain water—or at least go easy on the use of soap. Perspiration from the apocrine glands under the arms and in the vaginal area produces body odor as a result of bacterial activity, making it necessary to wash these areas daily. But since dry skin produces very little oil, it's rarely necessary to use soap over the entire body every day.

When too much soap is used on dry skin, the skin becomes inflamed, causing burning and itching. When this happens, it may be necessary to rub oil on the skin following a bath.

*Note:* Regardless of the type of skin you have, remember that after middle age your skin will probably produce less oil, requiring less wash-

---

how to make a cornmeal scrubbing paste

To use cornmeal as a scrubbing grain, mix about one-quarter cup cornmeal with enough warm water to make a paste. Let the mixture soak for awhile to reduce its coarseness. Apply the paste to your face and let it dry. Then rub it off with a dry washcloth. Follow this with a warm water rinse, then a cold water rinse.

You can rub cornmeal over your entire body when you want to glow velvety pink. Just take the wet cornmeal in your hand and rub yourself all over.

ing. So be sure to ease up on the use of soap when it seems to irritate your skin.

### How to Handle Inherited Dry Skin

If you suffer from *true dry skin*, or ichthyosis, which is an inherited skin disorder evident from childhood, you may not be able to use soap on your body during the winter. Oil and sweat glands are less active when the weather is cold. This allows dry winter air to evaporate moisture from your skin until it cracks from dryness. Air heated indoors is usually also dry, adding to your misery. You may find it absolutely necessary to rub olive oil (or a skin oil) on your skin after a plain-water shower. Or, you may rinse in a tub of fresh water that contains a small amount of oil.

Make sure that your diet contains adequate vitamin A and vegetable fat. It is well known that a deficiency in the essential fatty acids can result in dryness of the skin. If you want to help protect your children from developing skin problems, breast feed your babies. Human milk is rich in essential fatty acids, whereas cow's milk is rich in harmful saturated fat.

*Note*: Even if you have *normal* skin, excessive use of soap and hot water during the winter may produce a temporary but uncomfortable drying of your skin. Don't wash your skin any more than necessary to remove accumulated oil and dirt.

### Too Much Sun Can Age and Wrinkle Your Skin

The rays of the sun are responsible for more wrinkled skin than any other single factor. Even if your diet is rich in vitamins A and C, excessive exposure to the ultraviolet rays of the sun can damage the collagen that normally keeps your skin smooth and elastic. This does not mean, however, that you should stay out of the sun completely. You need a certain

---

**moisturizing oil bath**

Put a few tablespoons of olive oil into a tub of fresh, warm water. Stir the water to mix in the oil. Lie down in the tub so that your entire body is covered by the water and soak in the water for several minutes. When you get out of the tub, pat yourself dry so that a thin film of oil will remain on your skin. The oil will help your skin hold the mositure it has absorbed, and it will help protect against the drying effect of winter air and heated buildings.

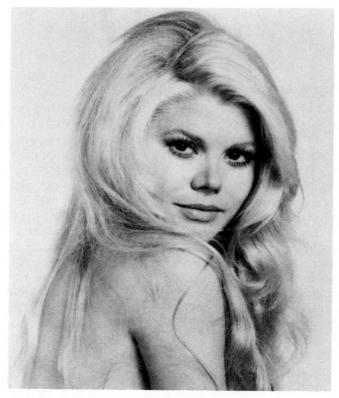

*Television star Charo keeps her skin smooth and youthful
by avoiding excessive exposure to the sun's rays*

amount of exposure to the sun's rays for vitamin D and for good skin tone. But you must be careful to avoid overexposure. A sunburn is very damaging to the deep tissues of the skin.

### Tan Your Skin Gradually

If you want a suntan rather than a burn, it's very important to tan yourself *gradually* so that your skin will have a chance to protect itself against the penetrating ultraviolet rays. Once your skin has tanned and thickened, less damage is done to the deep collagen fibers during prolonged exposures to the sun. It's best, however, not to stay in the sun any longer than required to maintain a *light* tan. Baking in the sun day after day to maintain a dark tan will age your skin so rapidly that you'll look 20 years older than you really are when you pass middle age. Your chances of developing skin cancer will also be greater. Skin that has been overexposed to the sun's rays for several years may be disfigured by dilated blood vessels, splotchy pigmentation, and warty, brown growths.

To make sure that you don't damage your skin with too much sun in acquiring a tan, start with a 15-minute exposure on each side of your body. Increase the exposure time by five minutes each day until you get the degree of tanning you want or until you reach a two-hour exposure. You should *never* stay in the sun longer than two hours! Try to stay out of the sun completely between 11 a.m. and 2 p.m. when the sun's rays are strongest.

Remember that the ultraviolet rays of the sun can still reach your skin on a cloudy day. Never sunbathe for more than a few hours, even if the sun isn't constantly visible.

## What About Sun Tan Lotions?

If you use a commercial sun-screening agent on your skin, select one that contains para-amino-benzoic acid (PABA). An oily sunscreen is best for persons who do not have acne or very oily skin. Sesame seed oil will screen out about 30 percent of the sun's ultraviolet rays, olive oil about 20 percent. Any type of vegetable oil will help protect against sunburn. Mineral oil and baby oil (even when mixed with iodine) do *not* have any

---

### how to relieve sunburn

If you do get a sunburn, you can relieve the pain simply by soaking in a tub of cool water. Badly burned or irritated skin can be soothed with a tepid oatmeal bath.

Put three cups of cooked oatmeal into a cheesecloth bag and squeeze it several times in a tub of tepid water. Soak in the water for 10 to 30 minutes. When you get out of the tub, pat yourself dry so that a thin film of the oatmeal starch will remain on your skin.

Oatmeal water is often used to clean skin that is too badly irritated to withstand washing with soap. You simply pat your skin with an oatmeal bag while sitting in a tub of water. (You can use cooked oatmeal or you can purchase oatmeal powder from a drug store.)

*Note:* The best way to relieve the pain of an isolated burn is to apply cold, wet cloths directly over the burn.

sun-screening qualities and will *not* promote tanning or protect you from sunburn.

### Don't Neglect Your Nails

Your fingernails, like your skin and your hair, are primarily composed of protein, and their condition is determined largely by your nutritional status. An iodine or protein deficiency, for example, can result in brittle nails. The condition of your nails, like the condition of your skin, can reflect the presence of disease. Nails that are concave (like spoons) are often associated with chronic anemia. Blue nails may result from an oxygen deficiency caused by a heart or circulatory disorder, and so on. If your nails appear to be abnormal, show them to your doctor. In the meantime, remember that if you want to be assured of having strong, beautiful nails, you must eat properly.

### *How to Strengthen Your Nails with Gelatin*

No one knows why gelatin helps nails, since it is deficient in cystine, an amino acid known to be essential in the formation of nails. Practical experience and several scientific studies, however, indicate that gelatin does indeed strengthen brittle nails.

Each day, take seven grams (about one-quarter ounce) of unflavored gelatin in orange juice or water. Any improvement in your nails should become evident in six to eight weeks.

Although gelatin is an incomplete protein, it can combine with other sources of protein if taken with meals. Taken alone, gelatin might help your nails, but it will not satisfy your dietary requirements for protein. So don't let anyone talk you into going on an orange juice and gelatin reducing diet.

### *How to Handle Dry Nails*

Exposure to detergents and harsh cleaners and application of nail polish remover, nail hardener, or other cosmetics can dry or injure nails. If you have a problem with your nails, don't put anything on them but water and oil until you find out what is causing the problem. Soak your nails in water for several minutes and then rub them with vegetable oil to hold in the absorbed moisture.

## How to Clean Your Nails Properly

When you clean dirt from under your nails, don't use a sharp or metallic object. If you scratch the undersurface of your nails, the scratches will collect dirt that is difficult or impossible to remove. Clean your nails with a plastic or wood strip *after* you have soaked them in soapy water. Use an emery board rather than a metal file when you file your nails. Keep the cuticle pushed back with an orange stick so that you won't have to resort to use of chemical cuticle removers that might damage your nails.

Any manicurist can tell you how to groom your nails. Remember, however, that if your nails are unhealthy because of a nutritional deficiency, it will be difficult or impossible to make them beautiful.

## Give Your Toenails a Little Attention

Thickening of nails on the toes, especially the big toe, is common among women as a result of wearing tight shoes. The pressure of the shoe against the nail does not allow the nail to grow outward, forcing it to increase in thickness. If the pressure on the nail is not relieved, the enlarging nail may exert enough pressure on the nail bed to cause loss of the nail or an ingrowing nail.

Keep your toenails trimmed straight across and then make sure that your shoes don't squeeze your toes. Don't wear pointed, high-heeled shoes except on special occasions, and then for only a short period of time.

Deformed, corn-ridden feet with thick, ugly nails can shatter the aura of your beauty when you undress for your man. So it's important to wear properly fitted shoes. See a podiatrist if your feet begin to show signs of developing corns, bunions, or other problems.

## What to Do About Facial Hair

Facial hair is an unfortunate problem for some women, especially after the age of forty. When hair on the upper lip and chin is thick and dark, it is probably best removed by electrolysis. A small amount of hair on the upper lip or the face can often be concealed satisfactorily by bleaching it.

## Removal of Hair by Electrolysis

Permanent removal of hair by electrolysis (with an electric needle) may take many months since it is a slow and tedious process. It may take half an hour, for example, to remove only a few dozen hairs, and treatments may be spaced several days apart. Improper technique in electrolysis can result in pain and scarring, so be sure to consult a dermatologist for expert performance of this procedure.

### Eyebrow Plucking

Most women pluck their own eyebrows. This can be done quite safely if the skin and the tweezers are sterilized with alcohol before and after plucking. It's best to pluck only a few hairs a day (in a symmetrical pattern) so that you can watch for signs of infection. If plucking is painful, you can first numb the area by rubbing it with an ice cube.

*Note*: Plucking a hair from a mole or a wart could result in serious bleeding. Always use scissors to clip hair from a growth, even if you must clip it often.

### Wax Depilation

Fine, downy hair on the face can be removed quite easily with wax depilation. This can be done at home or in a beauty salon. A special wax is melted and applied over clean, powdered skin with a spatula. A strip of cheesecloth is pressed into the soft wax. When the wax hardens, the cloth and the wax are ripped off rapidly, pulling against the direction in which the hair is growing. This pulls the hair from its roots. The treatment must be repeated about every three weeks. Have this procedure done in a beauty salon or in a dermatologist's office before trying it yourself.

### How to Remove Body Hair

Hair growth over the body of a woman is not usually a problem unless

---

a formula for bleaching facial hair

If you have light skin and you want to conceal a small amount of facial hair by bleaching it, try this formula.

Mix two tablespoons of six percent peroxide with 15 drops of ammonia and one tablespoon of pure soap flakes. Apply the mixture to your face with a cotton swab, leave it on for 30 minutes, and then rinse it off with cool water.

there is a hormonal disturbance. It's quite normal, however, to have a heavy growth of hair under the arms and on the legs.

## Leg Shaving

The best way to handle hair growth on the legs is simply to shave it daily with an electric razor. Chemical depilatories can result in allergic reactions and require more time than shaving. Contrary to popular opinion, shaving does *not* cause hair to grow back thicker and darker. If you shave your legs with a razor blade, lather your legs with soap or shaving cream, use a sharp blade, and shave *against* the direction of hair growth.

## Underarm Hair Removal

The only safe way to remove underarm (axillary) hair is to shave it with a razor or clip it with scissors. Since underarm hair collects bacteria and body secretions that produce a bad odor, it's always best to keep this area as clean of hair as possible.

Female underarm hair is frowned upon in our society, and a strong underarm odor is totally unacceptable. But don't worry too much about an honest, characteristic body odor that occurs in spite of a daily bath. A certain amount of body odor might even arouse the animal instincts in your man. In nineteenth century France, body odor was considered to be sexually exciting. The French poet Charles Baudelaire, who was planning to visit his mistress when he returned from a vacation, telegraphed her the following message: "Don't wash. I'm coming home tomorrow."

## SUMMARY

1. Proper cleansing of your scalp is essential for beautiful, manageable hair.

2. A vinegar or lemon rinse will remove the film that remains on your hair after washing it with soap and hard water.

3. Large, clogged facial pores should be cleaned with soap and water rather than with cleansing creams.

4. Wet oatmeal or cornmeal can serve as a substitute for beauty grains in rubbing away dead skin cells that obstruct pores and oil glands.

5. Wash oily skin as often as necessary to keep oil from accumulating in pores.

6. Excessive washing with alkaline soap will remove the skin's protective oils and acids and leave it more susceptible to infection and irritation.

7. Women with inherited dry skin may have to rub their body with oil following a plain-water bath.

8. Excessive exposure to the rays of the sun will age your skin prematurely and may contribute to the development of skin cancer.

9. The condition of your fingernails can reflect disease, a nutritional deficiency, or lack of personal care.

10. Unsightly hair anywhere on your body can be removed with appropriate measures.

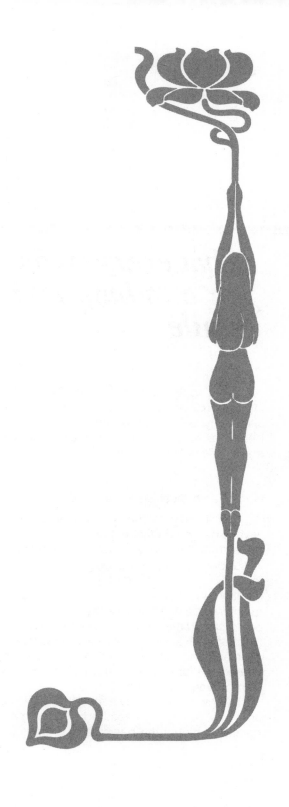

# what every woman must do for a radiant and healthy smile

Nothing detracts from female beauty more than bad teeth—and nothing is more permanent than *loss* of teeth. You can grow new hair and new skin, but you cannot grow new teeth. Since good teeth are as essential for beauty as for good health, this entire chapter will be devoted to the care and preservation of teeth.

### Good Teeth Must Be Maintained

Don't assume that just because you now have good teeth they'll always be good. Without proper care of your teeth and your gums, dental decay may flare up like a forest fire and creeping gum disease may result in sudden loss of teeth. Doctors used to believe that once a tooth has formed, its internal structure could not be influenced by good or bad nutrition. We now know, however, that good nutrition is essential for the maintenance of a firm, healthy tooth surface that will resist decay-causing organisms in the mouth. So even if you avoid use of sugar and brush your teeth after every meal, it's very important that your diet contain the vitamins and minerals your body needs to maintain a healthy tooth structure. Vitamin $B_6$, for example, may be just as important as calcium and vitamin D in preventing cavities.

Many nutrients play a role in maintaining healthy teeth and gums. The only way you can be assured of getting *all* of these nutrients is to eat a balanced diet of the basic natural foods (see chapter 2).

# Chapter 7

## How to Prevent Tooth Decay

Over 98 percent of the U.S. population is afflicted with tooth decay! This is undoubtedly the result of bad eating habits combined with inadequate cleaning of the teeth. Snacking on sweets and refined carbohydrates between meals, for example, or failure to clean the teeth after snacks and after meals allows the bacteria in the mouth to convert sugars and starches to powerful acids. These acids literally dissolve the calcium in the teeth to form holes where bacteria live and multiply. In areas between the teeth, under the gum margins, and in other sheltered or hard-to-clean areas decay may take place, unseen, at a rapid pace.

One of the first things you should do to combat tooth decay is to *avoid the use of sugar-sweetened foods and refined carbohydrates.* When you do eat such foods, you should brush your teeth afterward as soon as possible or at least rinse your teeth with water. Even if you eat honey, blackstrap molasses, and other natural sweets, you should still observe the same emergency cleaning procedures. In fact, sticky molasses may cause as much or *more* decay than sugar if it is not quickly removed from your teeth.

You should never fail to brush your teeth after a meal, and it's absolutely imperative that you clean your teeth before retiring for the night. Failure to clean your teeth after eating at night will allow bacterial activity to feast on sugar and food particles undisturbed for several hours. More damage is done to uncleaned teeth while sleeping than at any other time.

So even if you are tired, late getting in, or anxious to make love, you should not fail to clean and brush your teeth before you go to bed.

*Note:* Be sure to instruct your children in the proper care of teeth. The younger your children are when they begin to take care of their teeth, the better their chances of having beautiful teeth as adults. It's the responsibility of the parents to see that their children are properly fed and their teeth properly cleaned until they become old enough to assume responsibility for their own teeth. Once your children have acquired the habit of caring for their teeth as a result of your influence, they'll usually continue the care when they leave home.

### Gum Disease Can Result in Loss of Teeth

Although many teeth are lost to decay, the most common cause of loss of teeth is *gum disease*. After the age of forty, *gum disease accounts for more lost teeth than all other factors combined.* Three out of every four Americans suffer from gum disease, and almost 100 percent of all Americans over the age of 65 have gum disease. The result of all this is that one out of every eight Americans has no natural teeth, while about half of all Americans over the age of 55 have lost *all* their natural teeth. This is horrifying and tragic. But don't despair. If you're still young, or if you still have your teeth, there's plenty that you can do to keep them. In fact, with proper care of your teeth and your gums, and with adequate attention to your diet, you can *prevent* serious gum disease. If you already have bad gums, you can save your teeth and prevent further progression of gum disease by seeking specialized dental care and by following the self-help program outlined in this chapter.

Teeth properly cared for can be beautiful. Bad teeth can make you look like a witch. So, whatever you do, resolve now that you will give your teeth the attention they deserve. You owe it to yourself to avoid the pain, the expense, and the humiliation of losing your teeth.

### How Clara D. Saved Her Teeth

Gum disease, also called periodontal disease or pyorrhea, often goes on for years before it is detected or before obvious symptoms appear. This is one reason why it's so important to make regular visits to a dentist, so that he can catch the disease in its early stages. Many people, however, who have good teeth and no obvious dental problems do not visit a dentist.

Take the case of Clara D., for example. Clara had beautiful teeth with no cavities. "Why should I see a dentist?" she argued. "I don't need any fillings. And I brush my teeth regularly."

When Clara reached her 35th birthday, she began to notice that she frequently had bad breath. Her gums bled a little every time she brushed her teeth. She ignored occasional swelling of the gum around her back teeth. Eventually, a gum boil developed, and it was so painful that she made an appointment with a dentist. What he found shocked her. "You have pyorrhea," he said, "and we'll have to extract two of your molars to save the rest of your teeth. You'll also have to have periodontal surgery to get rid of the gum pockets around your teeth."

With the extraction of two teeth, expensive surgery by a periodontist, and an intensive oral hygiene program at home, Clara was able to halt the progress of the gum disease and save the rest of her teeth. But her teeth were never quite the same. Some loosening of her teeth and the installation of a permanent bridge made it more difficult to chew than before. She lived in fear of a recurrence of the infection.

Fortunately, Clara did a good job keeping her teeth and gums clean, and she did not lose any more teeth. Had she started earlier to use the cleaning procedures she now uses, she could have *prevented* the gum disease and the bone loss that loosened her teeth.

You can benefit from Clara's experience and take measures to save your teeth *before* trouble develops. All you have to do is follow the instructions outlined in this chapter.

### How Gum Disease Begins

There is normally a shallow crevice under the gum margin. If the teeth are not cleaned properly, a buildup of plaque and tartar in this crevice causes the gums to recede, allowing the buildup to creep farther and farther up under the gum margin. This irritates the gums, making them puffy, red, and shiny. Brushing usually results in bleeding, as indicated by pink toothbrush bristles. As the disease progresses, infection and bacterial activity in gum pockets literally eat away the bone around the roots of the teeth. If the disease isn't stopped, the teeth become so loose that they may actually fall out of their sockets. The bad thing about this disease is that it can often become far advanced before obvious symptoms appear. A careful examination is required to detect it in its early stage.

Although improper cleaning of the teeth is probably the major cause of periodontal disease, other factors may be involved. Malocclusion, or improper alignment of the teeth, for example, can loosen the roots of teeth, which can lead to detachment of the gums. Systemic disease or a vitamin deficiency can weaken the gums and contribute to the development of infection. A person who has diabetes may find it difficult to control gum infection. Calcium from the saliva and from tiny blood vessels under the gum margin builds up calculus more readily in some persons than in others, causing creeping detachment of the gums.

Obviously, periodontal disease can occur in some cases in spite of the usual cleaning procedures. When it does occur, heroic measures must be taken to stop it, and extensive cleaning procedures employed to control it. If you see a dentist regularly and you still have gum trouble, make an appointment with a periodontist. In the meantime, follow the cleaning procedures outlined in the remaining portion of this chapter. Remember that if you don't already have gum disease or loose teeth, use of these cleaning procedures will help *prevent* the development of trouble.

### How to Brush Your Teeth Properly

Until recent years, it was customary among dentists to advise their patients to brush *down* on their upper teeth and *up* on their lower teeth, *away* from their gums. And they usually recommended use of a *hard* brush. In modern dentistry, however, especially in the field of periodontics, these instructions are being changed. Now, instead of being told to brush away from your gums, you may be advised to *brush under the edge of your gums* as well as over all surfaces of your teeth. To do this, you must use a *soft* brush and angle the bristles in such a way that they slip up under the gum margin. Then, with short back-and-forth rotary strokes, you brush away food particles, bacteria, and other matter that tend to accumulate under the gum margin and between the teeth. If these deposits aren't removed, they feed the bacterial activity that decays your teeth and infects your gums.

### *Selecting a Toothpaste*

Since toothpaste is simply an abrasive that's used to clean and polish the teeth, almost any type of paste or powder that has abrasive qualities can be used as a dentifrice in cleaning the teeth. Powder is usually the most effective cleaner, since it contains more grains. Bicarbonate of soda, for example, makes a good dentifrice. Remember, however, that the more abrasive a dentifrice is, the greater the wear on your teeth. So be careful not to scrub your teeth so often or so vigorously with a highly abrasive dentifrice that you wear a groove in your teeth at the gum margin. Occasionally use only a wet brush to clean your teeth. You can purchase a special gum brush that is designed to be used without dentifrice. Ask your dentist for one.

Toothpastes containing stannous fluoride might be helpful in combating tooth decay by hardening the enamel of the teeth, especially for children.

*Note*: If you want to find out if you are cleaning your teeth adequately, you can chew a red disclosing tablet to dye your saliva. When you spit out the saliva, unclean spots on your teeth will show up as bright red stains. You can get disclosing tablets in any drug store.

### How to Clean Your Teeth with Dental Floss

Even if you brush your teeth after every meal, you should clean your teeth with dental floss at least once a day. If you don't use floss to remove food particles that are lodged between your teeth, tiny pinholes of decay may develop and go unnoticed until bacterial acids have penetrated deeply into the affected teeth. It's very important to use dental floss to remove plaque formation under the gum margins between your teeth (which cannot be reached with a brush). Since it takes about 24 hours for a sticky, invisible plaque to form on the teeth, it probably isn't necessary to use floss more often than once a day. If plaque isn't removed at least once every 24 hours, however, it may harden and become more difficult to remove.

The best time to use dental floss is at the end of the day just before retiring and after you have brushed your teeth. Just slip the floss up and down each side of each tooth several times until the floss squeaks. Remember that what you're trying to do is rake off a buildup of invisible plaque on your teeth. *Unwaxed* floss is best for this purpose.

*Be sure to slip the floss up under the gum margin on each side of each tooth.* Failure to do this would allow a buildup of plaque *and calculus that cannot fail to result in gum disease.*

*Note*: If your teeth are close together, it may be necessary to use a carefully controlled sawing motion to get the floss between your teeth. Using force to snap floss into the space between your teeth could injure or cut your gum, so be careful. Visit a dental hygienist for a professional cleaning and ask for a demonstration of how to use dental floss.

### How to Wash Out Gum Pockets with an Oral Irrigation Device

If you have periodontal disease with pocket formation under the edges of your gums, it's absolutely imperative that you keep these pockets washed out with an oral irrigation device if you want to save your teeth. Even if a periodontal surgeon has cut away the large pockets, you won't be able to keep your gums clean without irrigating them regularly.

You can purchase an oral irrigation device in any drug store. To use it, all you have to do is direct a tiny, pulsating stream of water up under your gum margins to wash out crevices and pockets. You'll be surprised at the amount of garbage you can wash from under your gums, even after you have brushed your teeth.

Food particles lodged in gum pockets can cause bad breath very quickly. *So be sure to use your oral irrigation device after every meal.* Regular use of the device can make the difference between keeping your teeth or losing them if you have pyorrhea or periodontal disease. It can also help *prevent* periodontal disease. Everyone should use an oral irrigation device, even when there is no apparent problem. To make sure that your gums are clean and healthy, and your breath fresh and sweet, try to make oral irrigation as much a part of your oral hygiene as regular brushing.

### How Karen Got Rid of Her Bad Breath

Karen T. had a terrible case of bad breath. She had noticed that her breath had a bad odor every morning, but she didn't know that her friends could smell her breath four feet away. She wondered why people often recoiled when she talked with them. When someone finally told her that something was wrong with her breath, she avoided close contact with people. She was constantly checking her breath, which was worse at times than others. Brushing her teeth didn't seem to help. Karen visited a dentist, who told her that gum pockets around her back teeth were trapping food particles that were decaying and feeding a bacterial infection. "This produces gas," he explained, "which is sometimes trapped in a pocket and then released all at once."

The dentist told Karen how to use an oral irrigation device and instructed her to get one immediately. After using the device for a couple of days, her bad breath disappeared completely! "My breath no longer smells bad in the morning," she reported. "And I can talk with people close up without offending them. The change in my breath is miraculous."

*Note*: Your tongue can also be a cause of bad breath, so be sure to brush your tongue occasionally if you want "kissing sweet" breath. The tongue is covered with a fleshy fuzz that catches food particles that can decompose to produce a bad odor. When your tongue appears to be coated, brush it with a toothbrush and then rinse your mouth with fresh water.

### How to Use Interdental Stimulators

Do you remember ever seeing grandpa or grandma break a twig off an oak tree for use in cleaning their teeth? They would chew the end of the twig until it was soft enough to press between their teeth and against their gum. Well, they had the right idea. Today you can buy scientifically designed interdental stimulators made of balsa wood. The wedge-shaped strip of wood is soft enough to press against the gum between your teeth so that you can stimulate your gums as well as clean your teeth.

Interdental stimulators are especially useful for cleaning your teeth when you dine out or when you are unable to brush your teeth. You can carry them around in your pocketbook just as you would a box of matches. A night club singer who has a habit of snacking between performances maintains that she can clean her teeth better with interdental stimulators than with a toothbrush. "When I'm singing over someone's table," she explains, "I have to make sure that there are no food particles in my teeth that could suddenly come loose and fly out of my mouth. It has happened, but not since I've been using those balsa wood toothpicks."

*Note*: The little rubber tip on the end of a toothbrush handle was designed for use as an interdental stimulator, but it is not as effective or as convenient as a balsa wood stick.

### Have a Dentist Scale Your Teeth Occasionally

No matter how good a job you do cleaning your teeth, you should see a dentist periodically so that he can scrape away tartar or calculus deposits in hard-to-clean spots around your teeth. The back sides of your upper and lower molars, for example, all the way back in your mouth, are very difficult to clean. If you have an excessive amount of calcium in your saliva, you may find it difficult to prevent a buildup of calculus behind your lower front teeth.

When deposits under your gum margins are especially bad, a dentist may find it necessary to deaden your gums with an anesthetic to permit a thorough scaling. Remember that it's practically impossible to take the best possible care of your teeth without professional help. The lives we lead and the foods we eat do not offer natural protection for our teeth.

### Don't Clench Your Teeth

Stop for a moment and think: Have you been clenching your teeth while reading this chapter? Do you have a habit of clenching your teeth when you are nervous or when you sleep? If you do clench your teeth, you must make a special effort to break the habit. Persons who habitually clench or grind their teeth often loosen their teeth so badly that they develop periodontal disease in spite of scrupulous oral hygiene.

The periodontal membrane that surrounds the roots of the teeth normally allows the teeth to move a little so that no strain will be placed on the roots while chewing. But when the teeth are constantly jammed into their sockets by habitual clenching, the membranes become damaged and bone around the roots of the teeth is absorbed. If the clenching is continued, the wobbly teeth detach from the gums and infection begins.

It's not likely that you'll be placed under the type of stress that some stars and celebrities must endure day after day. If you catch yourself clenching your teeth in everyday life, however, remember that if you don't quit it you may eventually lose your teeth.

### *Chew on Raw Fruits and Vegetables*

Chewing on raw fruits and vegetables is a good way to strengthen your teeth. If you like to snack between meals, or if you have a habit of clenching your teeth, keep a supply of fruit or vegetable sticks on hand to chew on. Carrots, celery, apples, hard pears, raw sweet potatoes, or turnip roots, for example, can be cut into sticks. If you're on a reducing diet, you may find these sticks especially helpful in satisfying your urge to eat something.

### Special Dietary Measures for Periodontal Disease

*Prevention* is always best when it comes to preserving your teeth. It's never too late, however, to improve your diet in combating gum disease. Supplement a good diet with at least 1,000 milligrams of vitamin C daily in divided doses. About 300 to 500 milligrams three times a day, for example, will speed healing of diseased gums. From 15,000 to 30,000 units of vitamin A daily, in divided doses of 5,000 to 10,000 units each, might be helpful in combating infecting. Although it's not likely that bone destroyed by periodontal disease can regenerate, you should make sure that you are not losing bone because of a mineral deficiency. Take at least two 10-grain bone meal tablets with each meal. Turn back to chapters 4 and 5 and study the material relating to bones and teeth.

Be sure to cut down on the sugar in your diet when you have gum disease. A high blood sugar feeds the bacterial infection in the pockets of your gums, making it difficult or impossible to control the infection.

## SUMMARY

1. Bad teeth can detract from physical beauty as well as result in much pain, expense, and embarrassment.

2. The two major causes of tooth decay are excessive use of sugar and refined foods and lack of adequate cleaning.

3. After the age of forty, gum disease accounts for more lost teeth than all other factors combined.

4. Failure to remove deposits accumulating under the gum margins is a major factor in the development of gum disease.

5. It's very important to brush your teeth after every meal and to use dental floss at least once every 24 hours.

6. An oral irrigation device is absolutely essential in cleaning out gum pockets that form in periodontal disease.

7. When you are unable to brush your teeth after eating, wash your teeth with water and then clean them with an interdental stimulator.

8. Be sure to see a dentist once or twice a year so that he can scrape away the tartar or calculus that accumulates around hard-to-clean teeth.

9. Remember that improperly aligned teeth or habitual teeth clenching can result in periodontal disease in spite of good cleaning.

10. When your gums are infected and you are losing bone in periodontal disease, supplement your diet with vitamin C, vitamin A, and bone meal.

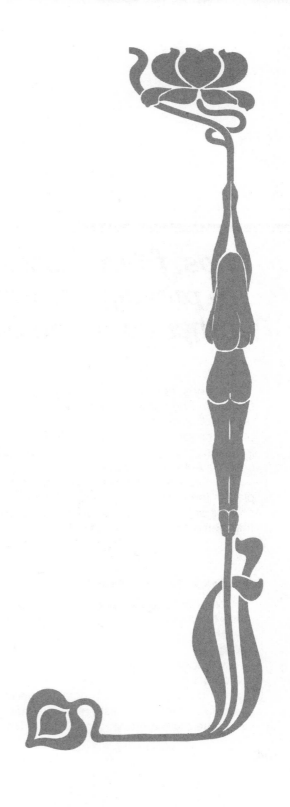

# tips from successful models to prevent cellulite and other common body problems

Every successful model knows how to keep her body slim, trim, and beautiful. She knows what to do about cellulite, a flat chest, bony shoulders, a double chin, flabby muscles, poor posture, sagging buttocks, and other common body problems. You don't have to be a model to benefit from the physical beautification procedures that models use, and you don't have to be a model to look like a model.

In this chapter you'll find solutions to many of the problems that plague the body of the average woman. Take care of your body the way professional models do and you'll be able to eliminate the trouble spots that detract from your physical beauty.

### How to Get Rid of Cellulite Forever

Women have always complained about lumpy deposits of fat around their hips and thighs. No one ever gave this fat a name, however, until a Frenchman published a book on the subject of "cellulite" in the early 1900s.

Although cellulite (pronounced "sell-you-leet") is still not mentioned in medical books, it is the subject of much discussion in the beauty spas of America. Some beauty specialists believe that cellulite is an accumulation of fat, water, and waste products that are *trapped* in scarred connective tissue compartments. The Federal Trade Commission recently issued

# Chapter 8

a statement to the effect that there is no such thing as cellulite and that advertised treatments for cellulite are therefore fraudulent. No one can deny the presence of the lumpy tissue referred to as cellulite, however. And it is a big problem among women who are sensitive about their physical appearance.

Most doctors feel that lumpy fat is the result of ruptured fat cells. This means that cellulite could probably be *prevented* with good nutrition and proper exercise. It is well known, for example, that vitamin C strengthens the collagen that holds tissue cells together. Vitamin E helps reduce scar-tissue formation that results from inflammation or injury. A nutritious, low-calorie natural foods diet helps prevent the engorging and rupture of fat cells. Preventing the development of obesity in childhood actually helps prevent the formation of *extra* fat cells. If you do not now have any lumpy fat on your body, then perhaps you've been living right. When lumpy fat does appear, there's plenty that you can do to improve your physical appearance. You might even be able to get rid of the fat so that your body will once again be smooth and beautiful.

*Note*: The lumpy fat called cellulite should not be confused with isolated tumor-like deposits of fat called "lipomas," which must be removed surgically.

Tissue that is inflamed or painful should be brought to the attention of a doctor. Cellulitis, or inflammation of connective tissue, is not the same as cellulite and should be treated by a physician.

### How to Prevent or Eliminate Cellulite

The first step in the treatment and prevention of cellulite is to reduce excess body fat. Once engorged fat cells have ruptured and become deformed by scar tissue, however, diet alone may not be enough to smooth out the lumpy tissue. After you have reduced all the excess fat on your body, you'll have to develop the underlying skeletal muscles to tighten and mold the overlying fatty tissue so that the fat will no longer appear lumpy. Remember that it's natural and desirable for every woman to have an outer padding of fatty tissue if she is to be soft, cuddly, and voluptuous. Without adequate muscular development to mold this fat, however, the body will not have the fullness and the contours that make the female figure beautiful. So while you need to reduce *excess* fat, it is neither desirable nor possible to eliminate *all* of the fat. It's absolutely impossible to mold fat properly—to eliminate uneven bulges—without taking adequate exercise.

Here are some important basic rules for every woman concerned about the problem of cellulite.

**1. Reduce excess body fat with a combination of diet and exercise.**   The reducing diet outlined in chapter 2 and the progressive resistance exercise program described in chapter 9 will provide you with an effective anti-cellulite program. Remember that diet alone will not get rid of cellulite. You must also exercise to *force* burning of stored fat for energy. And you must exercise *regularly* so that remaining lumpy fat will be smoothed and molded by the contours of well-developed muscles. Reducing body fat without developing the skeletal muscles may only allow residual fat and loose skin to sag grotesquely.

Women often complain that their lumpy fat looks worse when they go on a diet and lose weight. June C., for example, was a divorcee who developed a renewed interest in improving her physical appearance when she moved from a midwestern state to a coastal town. She lost 28 pounds on a popular reducing diet, but she complained that her hips and thighs were lumpier than ever. "My entire purpose in reducing my weight was to look better in a bathing suit," she lamented, "but I believe I look worse now than when I was heavier."

June was given a couple of exercises and advised to do them every other day for at least six weeks. After only four weeks she reported that her hips and thighs looked much better. "My thighs are rounder and much smoother," she observed, "and my hips look 100 percent better. The exercise obviously helps."

Exercise *does* help. It can make the difference between success and failure in developing truly beautiful hips and thighs.

Models who reduce their body fat to a minimum know that without adequate muscular development they would literally be "skin and bones." This is why so many models now use barbells and dumbbells in their exercise program to develop their muscles. The day of the bony-thin model is past. Almost all beauty contest winners now have full, rounded figures that have been molded by muscle-building exercises. It's no secret that most men prefer full, curvy figures. With proper exercise, you can get rid of cellulite as well as improve your figure, so be sure to study chapter 9 carefully.

**2. Use massage and moist heat to stimulate circulation and to soften scar tissue.** You can't massage away fat, but you can use massage to work out the fibrous deposits that tend to accumulate in lumpy fat. Once these deposits have been softened by massage, the circulation of blood, stimulated by moist heat or exercise, tends to wash out the hardened tissue. Get a full body massage as often as possible, but do not try to substitute massage for exercise; you need both. (Massage should be gentle and not painful. Simple kneading of the lumpy areas is all that is necessary. Every time you take a bath, use soapsuds as a lubricant and massage your hips and thighs.)

Vitamin E improves circulation and protects cells from the destructive, aging effects of oxygen. It also reduces scar-tissue formation. Turn back to chapter 4 and review the material on this important vitamin. Try to take about 100 units with each meal.

**3. Strengthen cell membranes with vitamins A and C.** It is now well known that vitamin C strengthens the collagen that holds tissue cells together. Vitamin A is also essential in building healthy tissue. A deficiency in either of these vitamins, especially vitamin C, contributes to aging and the development of lumpy fat by allowing deterioration of tissue cells.

The nicotine absorbed from cigarette smoke (in the mouth as well as in the lungs) destroys vitamin C in the blood. It also interferes with blood circulation by constricting blood vessels. Medical research has revealed that the wrinkles or "crow's feet" around the eyes of smokers may be caused by impaired circulation that damages collagen in the skin. This is one more reason why you shouldn't smoke cigarettes if you want to be beautiful as well as healthy.

Try to take at least 1,000 milligrams of vitamin C daily along with 15,000 units of vitamin A. And, to make sure that an undetected nutritional deficiency does not result in rupture of fat cells, eat a balanced diet of fresh, natural foods.

**4. Stay healthy!** If you eat natural foods and exercise regularly, chances are you'll be healthy, and this will minimize your chances of developing cellulite. Unfortunately, the female hormone estrogen seems to have something to do with the formation of lumpy fat, since it is estrogen that is responsible for characteristic female fat. (Men who are castrated to slow the growth of prostatic cancer or those who are given estrogen sometimes develop cellulite.) Use of birth control pills may upset hormonal balance and disturb venous circulation to trigger the formation of cellulite. Unrelieved constipation may create enough pressure in the pelvis to interfere with venous blood flow in the hips and thighs. Excessive use of salt may force water retention in swollen, ruptured fat cells.

There are probably many factors known and unknown that can contribute to the formation of lumpy fat in the body. *Most of these factors could be minimized or eliminated with a complete health-building program.* This means observing *all* of the rules of building and maintaining good health. Preventing obesity, for example, must be accomplished with the kind of diet that supplies all of the nutrients your body needs to be strong and healthy. (See *Doctor Homola's Fat-Disintegrator Diet*, Parker Publishing Company.)

**5. Let your skin breathe!**   Many women who are overly modest tend to keep their body covered 24 hours a day. You can tell at a glance when skin has not been exposed to sunlight, air, and water in outdoor activities. The flesh is spongy and sickly white, with skin so thin that it cannot conceal the bluish veins lying just beneath the surface. Blemishes, pores, hairs, and lumpy deposits of fat are clearly evident on skin that is starved for attention. You already know from reading chapter 6 that too much sunlight ages the skin. A certain amount of exposure to sunlight, however, improves the appearance of the skin by giving it color, tone, and thickness. These changes will help hide cellulite and other unattractive skin conditions.

Exposing the skin to sunlight, air, and water will actually aid in the elimination of waste products that might play a role in the formation of cellulite. There are many skin diseases such as psoriasis that can be prevented or alleviated by exposing the entire body to a small amount of sunlight. So, while you should avoid damaging prolonged exposures that result in a dark tan, you should make an effort to participate in enough outdoor activity to maintain a *light* tan. Sunbathe nude whenever possible. You'll look better and your man will find you more appealing.

### Fat Pads Can Be Surgically Removed

If you have inherited unsightly fat pads or skin flaps that persist even when you aren't overweight, you might want to have the fat removed by a plastic surgeon. A woman who has such deposits of fat cannot get rid of them without starving *all* of the fat off her body. No woman wants to be skinny, however. Besides, most men prefer their women to have a certain amount of well-shaped body fat to enhance lovemaking. So the trick in being desirable as well as beautiful is to get rid of excess or unsightly fat without losing the fat that is responsible for shapely female beauty.

In the case of "fat-pad deformities," it might be necessary to consult a surgeon. But when the problem is simply overweight, you can get rid of excess fat and build good health in the process by following the dietary recommendations outlined in chapter 2. Then, with the exercise program outlined in chapter 9, you can literally mold your body into the best possible shape.

### How to Improve the Appearance of Your Bust

Once the fatty tissue in the female breast begins to sag, there's not much that you can do to restore the lost firmness. Proper support of the breast will help prevent further sagging. There is, however, much that you can do to strengthen and tighten the muscles underneath the breasts. And if you feel that your breasts are too small, you can actually enlarge them by developing these supporting chest muscles.

One of the most common complaints heard among models and other women who wear bathing suits and low-cut dresses is that the area *above* the breasts is too bony. In spite of well-developed breasts, for example, the collarbones and the ribs are much too visible. Peter Lupus Leisure Health World usually recommends a special exercise, the incline press, to develop the pectoralis minor, a muscle just below the collarbone. This muscle is usually undeveloped because it is used very little in normal activities. With the incline press, however, the pectoralis minor muscle thickens enough to cover the ribs and make the breasts appear higher and more evenly developed. Sagging is also minimized.

### *The Chest-Lifter Incline Press*

If you are a member of a spa or a gym where they have an incline bench and a rack of dumbbells, you should include the incline press in your workout. You can, however, do this exercise at home if you follow these simple instructions.

Tip a chair all the way forward so that the chair back forms an incline. Pad the back of the chair with a cushion or a pillow. Sit on the floor and lean back on the padded chair so that your upper body will rest at an

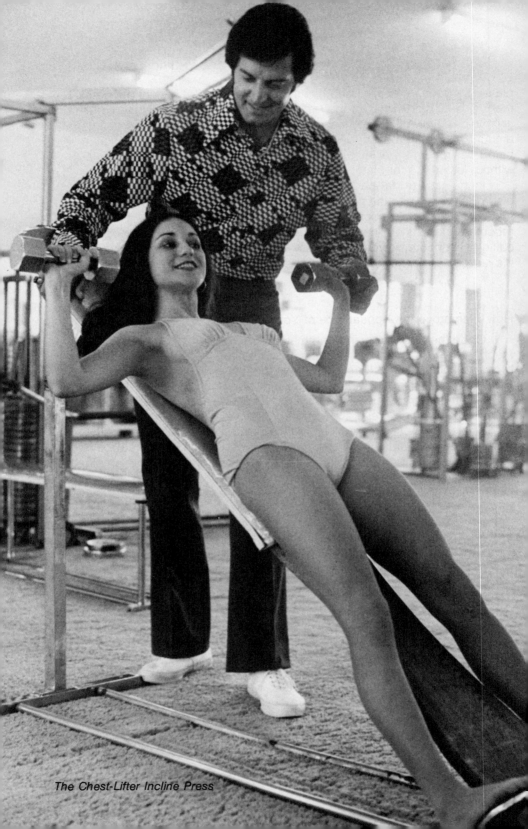

*The Chest-Lifter Incline Press*

angle. Hold a weight in each hand at shoulder level and press it straight up toward the ceiling. (See the photo.) Select a weight that you can press at least 10 times without straining. If you don't have any dumbbells, you can make up a couple of sandbags or use some other appropriate weight. You can purchase special bedroom dumbbells in most sporting goods stores. A pair of dumbbells weighing about 15 pounds each will be enough to begin with. Over a period of time, work your way up to as much weight as you can use for at least eight repetitions.

### The Breast-Enlarger Supine Lateral Raise

If you feel that your breasts are too small and you'd like to enlarge them a little, include the supine lateral raise in your exercise program. This exercise will develop the big pectoralis major muscles that lie underneath the breasts.

Lie flat on your back on the floor and hold a light weight in each hand at arm's length over your chest. Keep your arms straight (or your elbows slightly bent) and lower the weight to the floor on each side while inhaling deeply. (See the illustration.) Exhale while returning the weight to starting position.

Select a weight that you can use about 10 times without straining. Slowly increase the amount of weight you use as you grow stronger.

*Note*: You won't be able to use as much weight in supine lateral raises as in incline presses, so it will be necessary to use a different weight in each exercise.

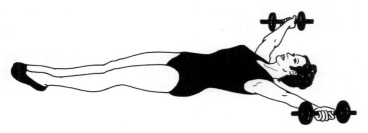

*The Breast-Enlarger Supine Lateral Raise*

### How to Eliminate a Potbelly

Vickie D. had a little potbelly that was clearly evident when she wore a bathing suit, and it was difficult to conceal when she dressed in revealing evening dresses. Since Vickie was not especially overweight, dieting was not the answer to her problem. "Every doctor I've been to has told me to exercise or do situps," she explained. "I simply cannot do situps. They hurt my back. One doctor recommended a special corset to flatten my stomach. But when I pull off the corset, my stomach pops out again. It's embarrassing to undress for my husband."

A quick examination of Vickie revealed a chronic back problem that made it impossible for her to do situps. Since her stomach bulge was largely the result of sagging abdominal muscles that had allowed her abdominal organs to fall, she was given a special exercise designed to reverse the condition. It took Vickie only about two months to correct a bulge that had been a source of embarrassment for several years.

If your abdomen shows the slightest sign of bulging in its lower portion, you should begin doing abdominal exercises immediately. Always check with your doctor to make sure that any *unusual* bulging is not the result of a ruptured abdominal wall.

### The Stomach-Flattening Incline Trunk Curl

This is the exercise that Vickie used to flatten her abdomen without hurting her back. It's also a good beginning exercise for persons who are too weak to do regular situps.

Fasten a strap around one end of a wide, thick board that's at least six feet long. Prop the strap end of the board up on a chair seat. Lie down on the board and anchor your feet under the strap. This incline position will help replace fallen organs as well as relieve compression on your spine.

*Curl only your head and shoulders up from the board.* (See the illustration.) Concentrate on contracting your abdominal muscles in each curl. Try to do at least 20 repetitions every other day.

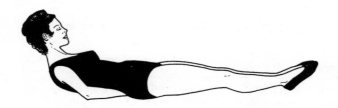

*The Stomach-Flattening Incline Trunk Curl*

*Note*: In this exercise, it's not necessary to sit up in order to exercise your abdominal muscles. Sitting up activates your hip flexors, which pull on your lower back.

If you prefer to do regular situps, keep your knees bent during the exercise in order to reduce the strain on your spine. You may, of course, do situps on the floor rather than on an incline board.

## What to Do About Sagging Buttocks

When a woman's buttocks are firm, rounded, and well developed, they are one of her most attractive features. Every man, when unobserved, steals glances at a female's hips. When a woman is shapely, she attracts a great deal of attention.

Models, stars, and other women who have shapely hips usually look good in a simple dress. When the buttocks sag because of flabby muscles, however, it is more difficult to dress attractively. And when corsets, coats, and other garments must be worn to *conceal* the hips, a woman loses one of her most valuable assets—at least from a man's point of view.

If your hips are so flabby that you have no shape in a pair of slacks or in a simple cotton dress, chances are bathing suits are out of the question. If you are a young woman, flabby buttocks can cripple your confidence in your physical appearance.

Since the buttocks are molded by the large gluteal muscles, there's plenty that you can do to lift them up and make them more shapely. The squatting exercises described in chapter 9, for example, are effective in shaping the hip muscles, especially when done with a barbell. If you want a simple exercise for your gluteal muscles, and you want to tone these muscles without enlarging them, do flat-footed squats while holding on to a bedpost. Or do the following hip-extension exercise.

### Buttock-Builder Prone Hip-Extender

Lie face down on the floor with both arms alongside your body and your hands palms up. Alternately raise each leg as high as you can. Be sure to keep your legs locked out straight so that your hip muscles will be forced to contract. (See the photo.) Do at least 10 repetitions with each leg, or as many as needed to tire your hip muscles. You should do this exercise every day whenever possible. As your hips become firmer and more shapely, you'll begin to notice the admiring glances from the men around you.

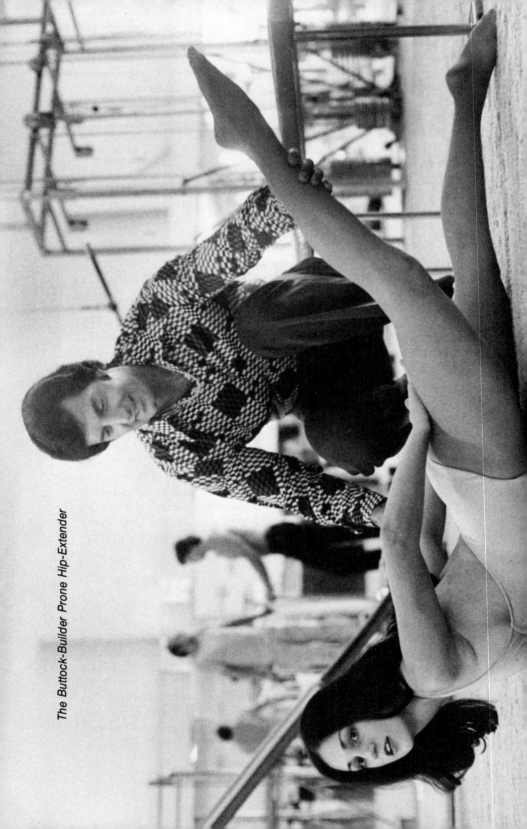

*The Buttock-Builder Prone Hip-Extender*

## How to Cope with Sagging, Wrinkled Facial Features

Facial wrinkles are often associated with aging. When a young woman's face begins to show wrinkles, it's usually assumed that she is aging prematurely. In most cases, the wrinkles could have been prevented! Wrinkles are rarely a true indication of aging. Cigarette smoking is sometimes associated with the appearance of wrinkles around the eyes. Excessive exposure of the face to the ultraviolet rays of sunlight can also wrinkle the skin by destroying the collagen fibers in the supporting layers of the skin.

Old people who have wrinkled skin on their face, neck, and hands often have smooth skin over other portions of their body. One reason for this is that the uncovered portions of the body are exposed more often to the rays of the sun, especially in the case of persons who spend a lot of time out of doors. If you're still young, try to protect your skin from constant exposure to direct rays from the sun.

A regular vitamin C supplement (1,000 or more milligrams a day) will help strengthen the collagen in your skin so that it won't sag prematurely.

## The Controversy About Facial Exercise

Some beauty specialists argue that once the collagen fibers in the skin have been damaged, facial exercises will increase the number of wrinkles by stretching the stiff and brittle collagen. Muscle tone is so important in preventing sagging of healthy tissue, however, that it might be best to include a little facial exercise in your beauty program. This can be accomplished simply by "making faces," or by contracting all the muscles of your face in every direction possible.

Muscles were made to be used. When they aren't used, they atrophy and sag. Weak, poorly developed facial muscles may result in uneven distribution of tissue around the bones of the face, spoiling the beauty of an otherwise lovely face.

## How to Erase Facial Wrinkles with a Facial Sauna

A daily facial sauna will help smooth wrinkled skin by softening damaged collagen and by increasing the moisture content of the skin. It might be especially helpful to take a facial sauna *before* doing facial exercises in order to lessen chances that muscle contraction will stretch stiff collagen fibers. Then, when the exercises have been completed, a small amount of vegetable oil rubbed on the face will keep the face smooth for hours by sealing in the moisture absorbed from the sauna. Turn back to chapter 6 and review the material on how to care for your skin.

### How to Use a Homemade Sauna

There are some expensive facial saunas on the market, but you can get much the same effect with a homemade sauna. All you have to do is place a pot of boiling water on a table, sit down in front of the pot, and drape a large towel over your head and the pot so that the steam will bathe the skin of your face. Don't get too close to the pot and be careful not to tip it over. If you're accident prone, and there's any possibility that you might burn yourself, shop around for an inexpensive but effective facial sauna.

After several minutes of a facial steambath, your skin should be plump and smooth from the effects of the moisture. This is only a temporary effect, but it might be useful before applying makeup for a date with your favorite man.

### What About a Face Lift?

If you have bags under your eyes or loose skin under your chin or on your neck, a good plastic surgeon can do wonders in lifting up the skin. In some cases, cosmetic surgery may be useful in maintaining the beauty needed to keep a job or find a man. Personality problems can often be eliminated by correcting facial features that are a source of embarrassment.

Whatever your reasons for considering cosmetic surgery, make sure that you do all you can to build and maintain a healthy body so that you won't be subjected to unnecessary or ineffective surgery.

### How to Be More Beautiful with Good Posture

No matter how firm or well developed your body might be, you can ruin your physical appearance with bad posture. We've all seen lovely women who appear to be flat-chested and potbellied because of bad posture.

Judith D. first realized that bad posture was distorting her chest and hips when she visited one of our offices for treatment of a backache. The simple postural exercise we re-commended to relieve strain on her spine improved her physical appearance so much that she rushed out and purchased a completely new wardrobe. "When you've got it, flaunt it!" she exclaimed with renewed confidence.

Judith did, indeed, look more attractive and more sexy. "I just cannot believe the difference in the attention I get from men since I have lifted up my chest with better posture," she confessed with astonishment. "Posture obviously has some-thing to do with sex appeal."

It's no secret that good posture emphasizes the natural beauty of the body. It also conveys a form of confidence that enhances personality as well as beauty. When posture is poor, it's virtually impossible to be truly beautiful and graceful. You've probably noticed that most models sit and stand erect, and they move about carefully and deliberately. Even when unrecognized, they attract attention with their regal posture. They sit and stand the way they do because they have developed the habit of protect-ing their body from damaging strains and ugly postures. They present themselves in the most attractive way possible—with good posture.

You can do the same thing. You can be attractive, graceful, and outstanding with good posture. You can look like "somebody" anywhere you go.

### How to Develop Good Posture

Developing good posture doesn't mean backing up to a wall and flattening your spine into a stereotyped posture. No two people have the same body structure, so don't try to stand exactly like someone else. All you have to do is *sit tall and stand tall*. Concentrate on maintaining an erect posture so that your spine doesn't sag. With a little practice you can learn to lift up your chest and hold in your abdomen with only a small amount of effort.

Remember that good posture should be a habit. If you try to sit and stand in such a way that excessive muscular effort is required, such posture would be too fatiguing to maintain. Throw away all the elaborate posture guides that require you to line up your ears with your ankles. Follow these simple instructions: *Sit tall, stand tall, lift up your chest slightly, hold in your abdomen a little, and then concentrate on moving about gracefully and effectively.*

## SUMMARY

1. Cellulite, or lumpy fat around the hips and thighs, can often be eliminated with a good diet, adequate exercise, and supplements containing vitamins C and E.

2. Resistance exercise to develop the skeletal muscles will mold body fat into a pleasing shape.

3. Isolated fat pads that persist after bodyweight has been reduced can often be removed surgically.

4. Sagging breasts are difficult to correct, but special exercises can be used to fill in bony areas above the breasts and to enlarge small breasts.

5. Trunk curls can be used to strengthen and flatten the abdominal muscles without placing a strain on the lower spine.

6. Sagging buttocks can usually be corrected by developing the gluteal muscles with special exercises.

7. Cigarette smoking, excessive exposure to sun, and vitamin C deficiency can result in premature aging or wrinkling of the skin by damaging its collagen fibers.

8. A facial sauna can temporarily smooth wrinkled skin by softening damaged collagen and by increasing the moisture content of the skin.

9. Cosmetic surgery, or a face lift, is sometimes useful in eliminating loose skin under the eyes and the chin.

10. Good posture makes you more beautiful by emphasizing the natural beauty of your body.

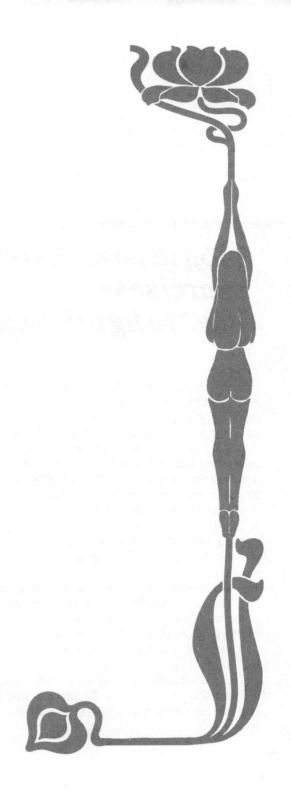

# progressive resistance exercises- key to figure tone

Until recent years, no one thought of using barbells and dumbbells to improve the female figure. Since men lift weights primarily to build big muscles, everyone just assumed that if a woman lifted weights she would look like a man. Fortunately, the physiology of a woman is different from that of a man. Female hormones *prevent* the development of large muscles. They also prevent the growth of facial and chest hair, and they are responsible for the delightful deposits of fat that make a woman's body beautiful and feminine. But a woman *does* have muscles, just like a man. And, with the exception of a few pelvic muscles, a woman's musculature is identical to that of a man's. This means that *both men and women can use the same basic exercises to develop their muscles*. The only difference is the amount of resistance employed and the amount of effort involved.

When a woman's muscles are well developed, her body fat is firmer and shapelier. Without muscles, body fat tends to sag; and in some portions of the body where there is normally very little fat, bones may protrude grotesquely. It is essential, therefore, that every woman have a certain amount of fat and a certain amount of muscle for a full, balanced figure.

Once excess body fat has been removed with a sensible diet (as recommended in chapter 2), progressive resistance exercise will tone and develop muscles that pad bony areas and shape the remaining body fat.

# *Chapter* 9

**How Ludelle Molded Her Figure After
Reducing Her Bodyweight**

Ludelle T. lost 28 pounds of body fat on a natural foods
reducing diet. Even though she had finally attained her
"ideal" bodyweight, she still wasn't satisfied with her physical appearance. Her flesh sagged, and her body was curi-
ously lumpy and flabby in spite of her thin-looking appearance. It was obvious that Ludelle's problem was flabby
muscles. Any further attempts to diet away the flabby flesh
would only reduce her to skin and bones.

Ludelle started a weight-training program to build her muscles. The results were miraculous. In six weeks her flesh was
firmer. In three months the saggy, flat areas of her body
began to appear more rounded. After several months of
regular training, Ludelle's well-developed body was attractive and appealing. "I look better now than I did 20 years
ago!" she exclaimed. "And I believe I even look younger."

It's never too late to improve your physical appearance by developing your muscles. In fact, the older you become, the more important it is to
exercise your muscles. Weight training offers the easiest and the most
effective muscle-building exercise available for men and women alike.

### Progressive Resistance Exercise Designed Especially for You

If you have a thin, bony body, flabby muscles, or a poor figure, your only hope of changing your physical appearance, as Ludelle did, is to exercise with barbells and dumbbells. No matter how weak you may be, you can adjust the resistance of each exercise to fit your needs. No other form of exercise can be so easily adjusted to the ability of the individual.

Every woman can use additional strength. Weight training is the ideal way to increase your strength while improving your physical appearance. Although your muscles will enlarge from regular use of the exercises described in this chapter, the enlargement will not be excessive. Women who already have unusually large hips, thighs, and calves in spite of reducing excess body fat may have an *inherited* body shape that cannot be changed significantly. Exercise can, however, result in an improvement in shape by toning muscles and by balancing muscular development. If your body is not symmetrical, you can, of course, concentrate more on developing those body parts that you feel need the most attention. All you have to do is pick the exercises you want to do for the body parts you want to shape or develop.

Both authors of this book have had extensive experience in weight training. Peter Lupus has won numerous awards for his perfect physique. Dr. Samuel Homola is the author of many books and articles on the subject of physical training. Both Mr. Lupus and Dr. Homola have instructed stars, models, female athletes, and housewives in weight training. Beauty contest winners as well as female athletes now lift weights to improve their physical appearance and to increase their strength.

In this chapter you'll get the best available instruction in weight training for women. Be sure to study this chapter carefully if you want to train safely and effectively with barbells and dumbbells (or "beauty bells") to improve your physical appearance. Female athletes who want additional guidance in weight training should read *Weight Training in Sports and Physical Education* (published by the American Association for Health, Physical Education, and Recreation, Washington, DC). Most spas now have weight-training facilities for women. If you don't like to exercise alone, visit your local spa for inspiration and encouragement.

---

**How a Hollywood Starlet Keeps Her Body Beautiful**

The lovely lady demonstrating the exercises in this chapter with Peter Lupus is Alexis Anne Alexander, a professional model and actress who uses weights regularly to keep fit. A winner of several beauty contests and a graduate of

Louisiana State University (majoring in drama), Alexis has appeared in a number of musical comedy revues and plays. The contours of her body show the beautiful, full curves of well-developed muscles.

"Before going on the Peter Lupus program," she testifies, "I was about 12 pounds overweight. Now, my weight of 102 is about right for my height of five feet, four inches."

Like most Hollywood starlets, Alexis takes a variety of supplements (along with a balanced diet) "to maintain my weight, keep up my stamina, keep my skin clear, and make my eyes sparkle."

Alexis does indeed sparkle, and she is a good example of the benefits of good nutrition and regular exercise. She works out at a California spa where she is also an instructor.

### How to Select the Equipment You Need for Weight Training

A *barbell* is simply a long iron bar with weighted discs on each end. You can adjust the weight of a barbell simply by changing the discs. Special locking collars hold the discs in place so that they won't slide off the bar.

When you begin your exercises, you'll use only the bar, which usually weighs about 20 pounds. As you grow stronger, however, you'll have to add weight to each end of the bar in order to make each exercise adequately resistant. Make sure that you have two 5-pound discs and two 10-pound discs. This will give you a total of about 50 pounds when you include the weight of the bar. You won't be using all of this weight in all of your exercises. But since you'll be using more weight in some exercises than in others, you'll have to have the graduated discs to be able to adjust the weight in the various exercises. Buy plastic-coated discs so that you won't have to worry about scarring the floor if you should happen to drop your barbell.

A *dumbbell* is a short, weighted bar that you can lift with one hand. (You use two hands to lift a barbell.) You can buy adjustable dumbbells, but you might prefer to use solid dumbbells so that there will be less danger of the discs sliding off the bar.

If you use *solid dumbbells*, you'll need two 5-pound, two 10-pound, and two 15-pound dumbbells—one for each hand. Select plastic-coated dumbbells in the color of your choice.

If you use *adjustable dumbbells*, you'll need two dumbbell bars, four 2½-pound discs and four 5-pound discs. With this selection of discs, you can adjust the weight of each dumbbell from five pounds to 15 pounds. If you do use adjustable dumbbells, *be sure to tighten the locking collars* so that the discs won't slip from the bar while you are exercising.

### How to Adjust the Resistance in Each Exercise

When you begin your barbell exercises, *use only the bar in each exercise for a couple of days* until you learn how to do all the exercises. Then, if you feel that the bar is too light to provide adequate resistance for your muscles, you can add five pounds to each end of the bar.

As you grow stronger, when you need more weight in some of your exercises, you can replace the 5-pound discs with 10-pound discs. You may then eventually add the 5-pound discs to bring the total weight to 50 pounds. Of course, you won't use the same weight in each exercise. And it's not likely that you'll use 50 pounds of weight in more than one or two of your exercises.

*It's very important that you keep your exercises comfortable, so that you won't have to strain to complete eight to 10 repetitions.* You don't have to meet a schedule in increasing the resistance of your exercise as male bodybuilders do. If you don't feel that you need any additional resistance, you don't have to add any more weight to the bar. The important thing is to do the exercises regularly and let your muscles take care of themselves.

### *How to Make Your Own Barbells and Dumbbells*

If you don't own a set of barbells and you don't have access to any, you can make your own with a broomstick and a couple of empty gallon-size plastic milk containers. All you have to do is put enough sand or water into each container to provide sufficient resistance. Each end of the broomstick may then be inserted through the handles of the containers to make a fairly good "barbell." As you grow stronger, you can increase the resistance of the exercise by putting a little more sand or water into each container. (Sand would be best, since it won't slosh around. Lead shot can be used for additional weight.)

You can use quart-size detergent containers as "dumbbells" simply by holding one in each hand.

With a little imagination, you'll be able to think of a variety of ways to make up weights for use in resistance exercise. For example, sandbags filled with lead shot can be used as dumbbells. Pails filled with rocks and

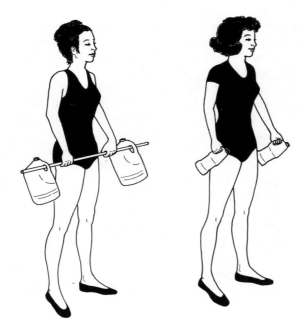

*Homemade barbells and dumbbells can be made
very easily by filling plastic containers with sand*

placed on each end of a notched pole can be used as a barbell. Heavier weights can be made by hardening cans of cement on the flattened ends of a section of water pipe. (See the illustrations.)

### Don't Exercise Too Much!

When you're overweight and you're trying to work off excess body fat, you should do calisthenic-type exercises in high repetitions every day. When you're lifting weights to improve your figure by developing your muscles, however, you should not exercise more often than every other day, especially if you want to *gain* weight. Three times a week, or Monday, Wednesday, and Friday, will be enough. You'll get *better* results with weight training if you don't exercise every day.

Actually, you won't have to work hard to get good results with weight training. In fact, chances are you'll *enjoy* doing your exercises. Just be sure to pick a time when you won't be disturbed.

### Picking a Time to Train

It really does not make much difference what time of the day you exercise as long as you are not pressured by other activities. If you want to exercise *comfortably,* however you should plan to exercise just before you eat or about two hours *after* you eat. It won't hurt you to exercise on a full stomach, but you might feel an uncomfortable pressure in your abdomen that will make you less than enthusiastic about doing your exercises.

If you don't want to do all of your exercises at one time, you can divide your program so that you can do a couple of exercises in the morning and a couple of exercises in the afternoon. Or you may do your upper-body exercises one day and your lower-body exercises the next day. It's okay to exercise with your weights a little each day as long as you don't exercise the same body parts two days in succession.

With a small amount of thought and planning, you can work a few minutes of exercise into your daily routine in such a way that your workout will not require any sustained effort.

*Note*: If you'd like your man to have more muscle, ask him to exercise with you. A man's muscles respond very quickly to progressive resistance exercise.

### How to Breathe When You Exercise

Since you won't be using heavy weights in your barbell exercises, you won't be straining enough to make breathing difficult. Just to make sure that you develop the habit of breathing properly, however, you should remember this rule: Always *exhale* during a heavy or prolonged exertion.

When you hold your breath during any form of exertion, contraction of muscles increases the pressure in your abdomen and your lungs, interfering with the return flow of blood to your heart. This may diminish the output of your heart enough to cause dizziness. So be sure to breathe rhythmically during your exercises. Never hold your breath!

### *Be Careful with Hyperventilation*

Breathing exercises are generally beneficial, but *excessive* forced deep breathing can be harmful. The best time to practice deep breathing is when you're breathless following exercise, when you need oxygen. If you hyperventilate, or deep breathe, when you don't have an oxygen debt, you may get dizzy from an imbalance in the amount of oxygen and carbon dioxide in your blood. Continued forced deep breathing can make you so dizzy that you might even lose your balance and fall.

Never prepare for an exercise by hyperventilating. Wait until *after* you finish your exercises and then practice deep breathing. Always stop forced deep breathing, however, when you begin to feel dizzy.

*Warning*: No matter what you have learned in yoga classes, never hyperventilate and then hold your breath while performing an exercise. Combining hyperventilation, breath holding, and exertion could result in a blackout and a serious injury.

## Advanced Training for Women

Basically, all you have to do for good results in weight training is to go through each exercise once. As you grow stronger, however, or if you want a little extra development in some part of your body, you can go through some of your exercises *twice*. In other words, after you have been exercising for a few months you can do *two sets* of an exercise, using the first set as a warmup for the second set. You may then use a little heavier weight in the second set, so that you have to work fairly hard to complete the recommended number of repetitions.

If you do go through each exercise twice, rest a few minutes before doing the exercise a second time.

As your muscles grow in size and strength to keep pace with the increase in resistance, the bony areas of your body will disappear. But don't worry. You won't look muscular or sinewy. Your muscles will automatically be covered by a thin layer of fatty tissue that is characteristically female in nature. This fat will add to the padding you need in the bony areas around your chest, shoulders, and back. Obviously, *weight training is a good way for a thin woman to gain weight without adding an excessive amount of fat.*

## How Nadine R. Gained 15 Pounds in the Right Places

Poor Nadine looked like a "bag of bones." She was so thin and underweight that people were constantly asking her if she had been ill. Nothing she did seemed to help her gain weight. "There are plenty of books that tell you how to lose weight," she complained. "Why can't someone tell me how to *gain* weight?"

Nadine did all five of the exercises described in this chapter. As her muscles grew, she began to eat more. She gained 15 pounds in nine months! And the muscle she grew was padded with new and firm feminine fat. "I feel more like a woman with a little meat on my bones," Nadine said with obvious satisfaction. "My husband says I certainly *look* more like a woman."

If a woman as thin and weak as Nadine can make such miraculous changes in her physical appearance, you can, too!

### What About Muscle Soreness?

Muscle soreness won't be a problem if you follow instructions and start out lightly in your exercises. As you begin to add weight to the bar, however, you might experience a little soreness in certain muscles. Since you won't be exercising more often than every other day, however, chances are you'll be over most of your soreness before it's time to exercise again. When you do feel unusually sore, a hot bath or a few calisthenics will probably relieve the soreness. Unless persistent soreness is excessive and results in pain during the performance of your exercises, it's okay to go ahead and work out. In fact, barbell exercises, in pumping blood through your muscles, will usually relieve soreness. So don't use a little soreness as an excuse not to do your exercises. Once you have become accustomed to exercising (after a couple of weeks), you won't get sore at all.

Remember that you may have to exercise regularly for about six weeks to see any visible changes in your physical appearance.

### Basic Barbell Exercises for Women

There are only five exercises that you have to do to cover all the major muscle groups of your body and they are all described in this chapter. If you don't want to do all of these exercises, you can do only those you feel you need most. For example, if you're heavy on the bottom and lacking up top, you can do only the upper-body exercises. If you have thin calves, you can do the calf exercise, and so on. Probably the biggest problem area among sedentary women is around the shoulders and upper chest, where muscular development may be so lacking that the shoulder blades, collar bones, and ribs are unhappily prominent. One or two barbell exercises will usually fill in these areas. If you have a generally poor figure, however, you should do *all* of the exercises so that you'll have beautiful, balanced proportions.

## Gripping the Bar

In all of the barbell exercises described in this chapter, you'll grip the bar in one of two ways: with an underhand grip or an overhand grip.

In the *underhand grip*, you lift the barbell from the floor with your hands *under* the bar; that is, with your palms turned up.

In the *overhand grip*, you grasp the bar with your palms turned down.

## The Upright Rowing Motion— For Shoulders and Upper Back

Stand erect with a close overhand grip on a barbell you're holding down at arm's length in front. Lift the bar up to your neck, pointing your elbows forward and up. (See photo 1.)

The upright rowing motion will develop the muscles on the front of your arm as well as the muscles around your shoulders and upper back.

If you want to do a *specific* shoulder exercise, you can do *dumbbell lateral raises*. You simply raise a pair of dumbbells from your sides to overhead, with straight arms, while standing erect.

### How a Top Model Added Attractive Padding to Her Shoulders

Christine P. was a gorgeous redhead who modeled expensive clothes in fashion shows. When she modeled strapless gowns, however, her shoulder girdle was conspicuously square and bony. "When my shoulders are uncovered I feel exposed and naked," she complained. "But I cannot allow myself to gain any more weight to cover those bones. My hips are already too heavy."

Christine was instructed in the use of two exercises: the upright rowing motion and the incline dumbbell press (see chapter 8), which she did faithfully. Six months later, she looked like a different woman in a strapless gown. "My shoulders now have a pleasing round slope," she reported gratefully. "I gained two pounds of shoulder muscle without

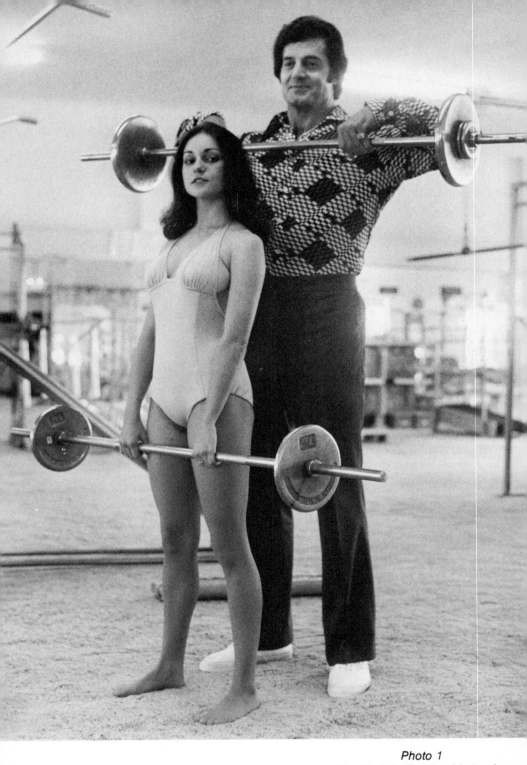

Photo 1
The Upright Rowing Motion for
Shoulders and Upper Back

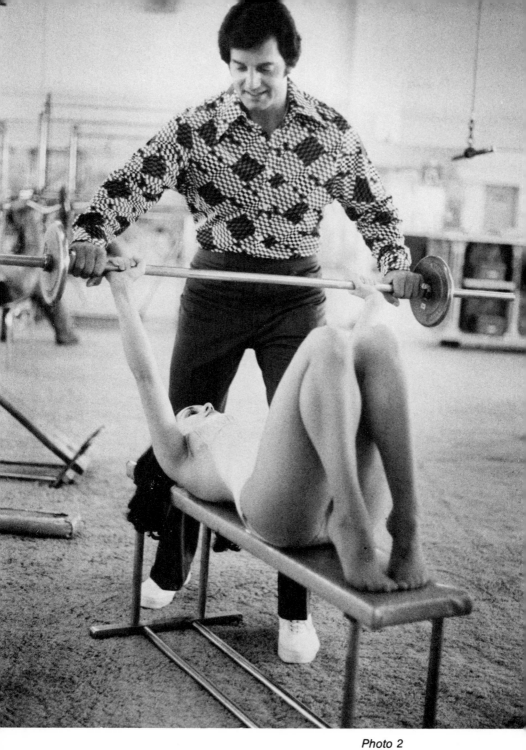

*Photo 2*
*The Chest-Building Bench Press*

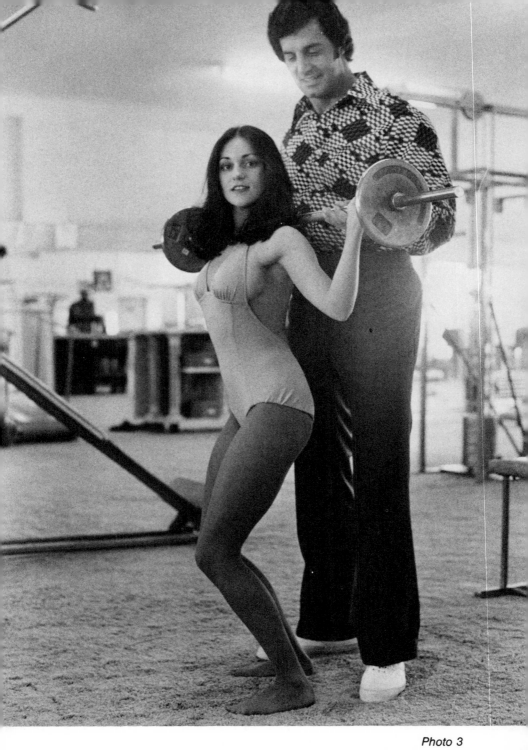

*Photo 3*
*The Barbell Squat for*
*Firm Hips and Thighs*

adding an ounce to my hips. My figure is much better balanced now. Thanks for the tip."

You're welcome, beautiful lady!

### The Chest-Building Bench Press

The bench press is a good exercise for developing the chest muscles that lie beneath your breasts, as well as the muscles on the back of your arm. This exercise is easy to do. After you have become accustomed to doing bench presses, you'll probably be able to use 50 pounds with no trouble at all.

Lie on your back on a low bench and press the barbell from your chest straight-up to arm's length. (See photo 2.) Have your man help you do this exercise—and be careful not to bruise your breasts.

If you have saggy breasts and your collarbones are unusually prominent, do the incline dumbbell presses described in chapter 8. Or you may simply do your bench presses on an incline bench.

### The Barbell Squat for Firm Hips and Thighs

If you can't do several full squats with only your bodyweight, practice the squat while holding onto a bedpost (see chapter 8) before attempting to squat with a barbell. When you are strong enough to begin squatting with a barbell, the added resistance will mold the muscles of your hips and thighs into beautiful, round curves.

To begin with, use only the bar in your squats. Place the bar across your shoulders behind your neck. Keep your head up, your feet flat, and your spine as vertical as possible while you squat. (See photo 3.) If you can't keep your feet flat on the floor when you squat, place a board under your heels. Remember, however, that *flat-footed* squats are best for the muscles of your hips.

### Straight-Arm Pullovers for a Deeper Chest

When you finish doing your squats, you should be breathing heavily. This will be a good time to do a breathing exercise. Even if your breasts are well developed, you'll be more impressive if your rib cage is lifted to deepen your chest and improve your posture.

If you don't have a low bench, lie on the floor with a cushion under your upper back. Hold a barbell bar or two light dumbbells at arm's length over your chest. (Use a shoulder-width overhand grip on the bar.) Lower the weight back over your head with straight arms while inhaling deeply. Exhale while returning the weight to starting position. (See the photo of the exercise to correct dowager's hump in chapter 12.)

Since the straight-arm pullover is primarily a breathing exercise, be sure to use a weight that's light enough to permit full expansion of your chest. The muscular contraction involved in the performance of this exercise will actually aid expansion of your lungs.

*Note*: If you use a bench when you do this exercise, don't try to lower the weight to the floor. Be careful not to place a strain on your shoulders.

### Heel Raises for Shapely Calves

Are your calves thin and straight instead of full and round? If so, the only possible way you can improve them is to do heel raises with a barbell.

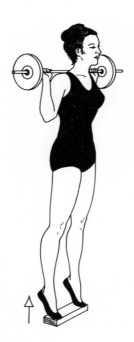

*The Calf-Building Heel Raise*

Stand erect with a barbell across your shoulders behind your neck. Rise up and down on your toes 15 times or more, until your calves begin to ache. (See the illustration.) Use as much weight as you can handle safely. If you prefer, you may simply hold the weight down at arm's length in front while you do heel raises.

When you become accustomed to doing heel raises, do them with the forepart of your feet resting on a thick board. This will allow you to drop your heels lower in order to stretch ankle tendons that have been shortened by wearing high-heeled shoes. (Short ankle tendons can cause backache!)

### How Laura Shaped Her Calves

The only flaw in Laura's figure was the shape of her calves. They were so straight and flat that they had no shape at all. With regular use of heel raises with a barbell, however, she added a full inch of muscle to each calf. "It took me six months to get that extra inch," Laura admitted, "but it was worth it. My calves look better and my stockings fit better. I no longer try to hide my calves by wearing slacks."

*Note*: Since the calf muscles are dense and tough, they are much harder to develop than the other muscles of your body. If you feel that you need larger calves, do your heel raises regularly for as long as it takes to get the improvement you want. Regular contraction of your calf muscles will also help prevent circulatory problems and leg cramps by pumping blood through your legs.

## SUMMARY

1. Progressive resistance exercise with barbells and dumbbells will improve your figure by developing muscles that mold body fat and pad bony areas.

2. Your female hormones will make it impossible for you to overdevelop your muscles.

3. In every exercise you do, make sure that the weight you use is not too heavy to permit eight to ten comfortable repetitions.

4. You can adjust the resistance in each exercise by changing the discs on the bar.

5. If you exercise indoors, use plastic-coated discs on your barbells and dumbbells.

6. It's not necessary to exercise more often than every other day to get good results with weight training.

7. Either exercise *before* you eat or about two hours *after* you eat.

8. Try to breathe rhythmically while you are doing a barbell or dumbbell exercise.

9. Weight training is ideal for the thin woman who wants to gain weight and improve her figure without adding flabby fat.

10. If you don't want to do all the exercises described in this chapter, pick the ones you need most.

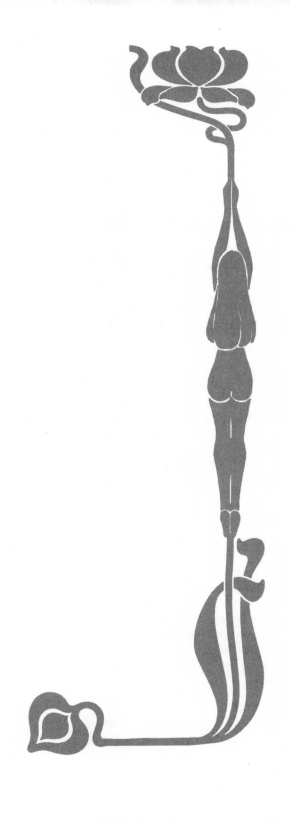

# how to be a sexually fulfilled woman

Are you a sexually liberated woman? If you aren't, your sex life may be hindered by inhibitions that stem from taboos and misinformation passed along to you from generations past. Did you know, for example, that at the turn of the century it was commonly accepted that women should not and could not enjoy sex! Sexual desire among women was, as one physician wrote, "a vile aspersion." Sex was a duty for married women to perform solely for the purpose of pleasing a husband and having babies. Women looked upon sex as an animal act that should be avoided whenever possible. It was unthinkable that a woman would desire sex, much less enjoy it. These Victorian standards were transmitted from well-meaning mothers to unsuspecting daughters.

It is tragic and saddening that so many women, influenced by puritanical authorities, have lived and died without fully enjoying the healthful pleasures of an active sex life. Even today, many adult women, schooled by misinformed parents, are unable to throw off the mental and emotional shackles that deprive them of a happy, guiltless sex life. Many young women in years past, influenced by puritanical mothers, were able to shut off their sexual desires so completely that they truly felt that sex for pleasure was a useless and disgusting activity.

## From Freud to Masters and Johnson

Sigmund Freud, in the 1930s, probably did more than anyone to help

# Chapter 10

women break away from notions that repressed their sexual desires. It was Freud who first recognized the harm being done to the health and the minds of women who were sexually repressed or who were guilt-ridden as a result of experiencing sexual desire. Even Freud may have been male-centered in his analysis of the situation, however, for he proposed the notion that a mature, truly feminine woman had a *vaginal* orgasm, which, of course, depended upon penetration by the male. Furthermore, when a woman had a vaginal orgasm, she was supposed to climax simultaneously with her husband. Clitoral orgasm, which could be brought about simply by rubbing the clitoris with the hand, was considered to be a practice of immature, less feminine women.

As a result of Freud's theories, there are husbands today who feel inadequate if they fail to bring their wives to a climax every time they have sexual intercourse. And there are women who are ashamed to admit that they cannot climax without clitoral stimulation. Many women who don't climax during intercourse often *fake* an orgasm to bolster the egos of their husbands. They may then be forced to masturbate secretly, or silently suffer from sexual frustration. Obviously, such a situation is likely to go uncorrected, depriving both the husband and wife of all the joys of sex.

The Kinsey survey, *The Sexual Behavior of the Human Female*, published in 1953, was the first major breakthrough in revealing the sexual plight of women. It was not until publication of the work of Masters and Johnson in the 1970s, however, that real progress was made in offering *solutions* for female sexual problems. As a result of their work, women are

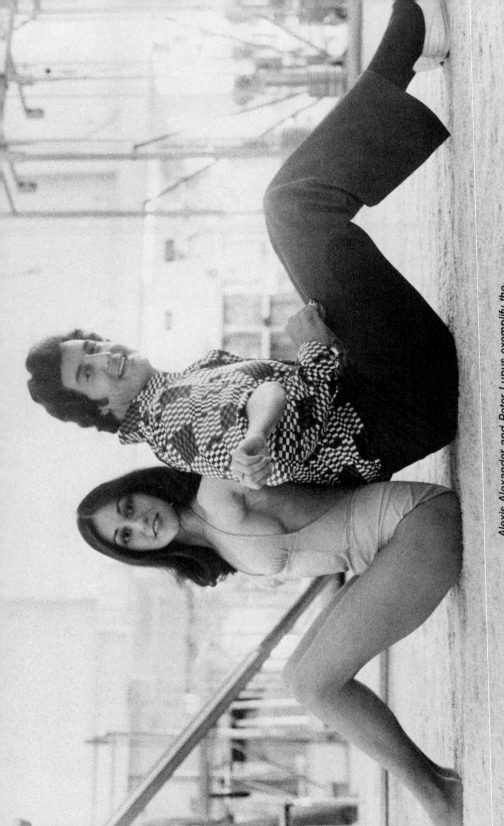

*Alexis Alexander and Peter Lupus exemplify the physical appeal that makes women and men sexually attractive*

finally being liberated from the misinformation and false standards that have so long deprived them of their full share of sexual pleasure.

### Men and Women Are Sexual Equals

Today, we know that every woman should be able to enjoy sex just as much as any man. There is really no difference in the desires and the pleasures felt by men and women. Sexual repression of women had only made it appear that women were less interested in sex. Males and females are different anatomically and emotionally, but their sexual needs are identical and should be satisfied equally.

### The Key to Female Orgasm

Regardless of what the followers of Freud believe, it is now well known that the clitoris is the nerve center of a woman's orgasm. Normally, penetration of a woman's vagina during sexual intercourse should be a pleasurable sensation that contributes to a sexual climax. But it is direct or indirect stimulation of the clitoris that brings a woman to orgasm.

### Clitoral Response

When a woman is ready and fully prepared for sexual intercourse, the inner lips of her genitals swell and become engorged with blood. The clitoris also swells, much like a man's penis. During intercourse, the clitoris may be stimulated indirectly by rhythmical tugging on the surrounding tissues or by direct contact with the penis. When the clitoris is fully erect, it points down toward the vaginal opening. If it is adequately exposed, it is more readily stimulated by direct contact or by pubic pressure.

As every woman knows, the clitoris is located at the top of the vaginal opening, at the junction of the inner lips. When it is erect, it may be from one-half to one inch long. Only the tip of the clitoris may be visible, however, as it protrudes from the surrounding tissues.

### Foreplay Helps Assure an Orgasm

Unfortunately, some women have difficulty getting adequate clitoral stimulation during intercourse. Since it generally takes longer for a woman to reach a climax, it is sometimes necessary for a woman to prepare herself (or have her man do it) with foreplay and manual manipulation of her genitals so that she will be ready and well lubricated before beginning intercourse. When the labia are congested, they'll grip the penis snugly so that an erect and sensitive clitoris can be stimulated indirectly by labial tugging.

Remember that it is nice but not absolutely necessary for a woman and her man to climax simultaneously. When you are making love with your man, you should concentrate primarily upon reaching your own climax. Then, when you do climax, the sounds and motions of your ecstasy will very likely bring your man to a climax. If you do not climax before he does, and you feel that you are approaching an orgasm, continue with him until you do climax. Most men can maintain enough of an erection to continue with intercourse for a short time after ejaculating.

Surveys indicate that the majority of men climax within two minutes after beginning sexual intercourse. So, if you tend to be slow in reaching a climax, you should try to get a head start with plenty of preliminary stimulation before allowing your man to penetrate you. With a little practice, your man can learn to prolong intercourse by holding back until you begin to feel the approach of your orgasm.

### The Problem of Intercourse without a Climax

If you fail to have an orgasm during intercourse, don't worry about it. Ask your man to bring you to climax by manipulating your genitals with his hand—or you can do it yourself while lying alongside him. If you're uncomfortable masturbating in the presence of your partner, ask him to masturbate with you occasionally. Show him the correct way to manipulate your clitoris. Mutual masturbation can provide exciting variety in your sex life, and it will help lower the barriers that inhibit your sexual response. It may also prove to be a convenient way to relieve sexual tensions when medical problems do not permit intercourse. When you do have to depend upon masturbation for orgasm, it's much better to share such pleasure with your man than to do it secretly.

### *Aids to Orgasm*

There is now considerable evidence to indicate that women who cannot climax during intercourse can often do so after practicing masturbation. An orgasm induced by masturbation may be more intense than an orgasm experienced during sexual intercourse, since masturbation permits more direct stimulation of the clitoris. But climaxing with a man in your arms may be more emotionally satisfying, so keep trying!

It's not unusual for some women to consistently have trouble climaxing during intercourse. In other words, they occasionally climax, but with considerable difficulty. If you have that problem, anything you can do to help you reach a climax with your man is okay. If you're turned on by oral sex, clitoral manipulation, a vibrator, use of mirrors, sex movies, or any other approach, don't hesitate to use it in preparing for intercourse. The important thing is to enjoy sex with your man without pressure, guilt, or embarrassment. If you still fail to reach a climax during intercourse, you should finish by whatever means you choose. It's always better to relieve sexual tension than to allow it to go unrelieved. Remember, however, that it's not absolutely necessary for you to climax every time you go to bed with your man. If you occasionally fail to experience enough response or desire to pursue an orgasm, you don't have to force yourself to a climax. You may simply wait until the next time.

### How Jeanette Achieved Her First Orgasm

When Jeanette T. and her husband made love, she enjoyed the attention but she didn't experience the thrill described by some of her friends. In fact, Jeanette admitted that she didn't think she had ever experienced an orgasm. No matter how hard she and her husband tried, she could not reach a sexual climax. And since she had never masturbated, she had no idea what an orgasm was like. Unfortunately, because of ego or ignorance, it had never occurred to Jeanette's husband that there might be other ways to bring her to a climax. Her strict training would not permit her to masturbate alone. "It would be sinful," she insisted.

A physician friend finally advised Jeanette and her husband to experiment together with masturbation. Jeanette experienced her first orgasm while masturbating during foreplay. Soon she was able to climax occasionally during intercourse. Her inhibitions were eventually replaced with a sexual aggressiveness that virtually assured an orgasm for her and an exciting time for her husband. Jeanette described her orgasms as "the most intense pleasure I have ever felt. It always leaves me relaxed, completely satisfied, and totally in love with my husband."

### Every Woman Can Climax

Most doctors now agree that there is no such thing as a truly frigid woman. Every woman is capable of having an orgasm. And a woman who can climax only with masturbation is certainly not frigid. A woman who has never experienced an orgasm, and who does not enjoy sexual activity of any kind, may have psychological problems that must be handled by a psychiatrist. When mental barriers are lowered and an effort is made to pursue sexual pleasure, the pleasure usually comes. It is, of course, sometimes impossible for a woman to completely erase all the inhibitions created by early Victorian training. When this is the case, it would be better to tolerate minor inhibitions, such as making love in a darkened room or under the bed covers, in order to avoid mental distractions that might prevent a sexual climax. No woman should be forced to indulge in a sexual procedure she is not ready to accept.

### Mutual Consideration Is Important

No matter how inhibited you may be now, or how you feel about sex, remember that there normally isn't any difference in the sexual needs and desires of men and women. You are entitled to just as much pleasure, just as many privileges, and just as much sexual variety as your man. As an equal, there is no reason why you cannot be just as aggressive as your lover in satisfying your sexual desires by whatever means you desire. When lovers have a mutual concern for each other in attaining sexual satisfaction, the pleasure of one partner greatly enhances the pleasure of the other partner. In fact, when two people are in love, the pleasure expressed by a partner is half the pleasure of making love! So it's important that lovers give and receive equally, with both fully expressing the pleasure they are feeling.

### Sex without Love

If you deeply love your man, sex will be better. In fact, you'll probably never experience anything more beautiful, satisfying, or exciting than uninhibited sex with a man you truly love. But if you feel that you do not love your man and that you're stuck with him, there is no reason why you cannot obtain physical satisfaction from your relationship with him—unless, of course, he turns you off because he is mentally or physically repulsive to you.

It's nice to have sex with someone you love, but you should be able to relieve sexual tension on a purely physical basis, without any emotional attachment whatsoever, just as you do when you masturbate alone. And if you enjoy sexual intercourse, you'll experience more complete relief with a man you don't love than if you masturbate alone. Besides, many women admit to having fantasies during intercourse. Some imagine that they are in the arms of a favorite male celebrity. And they confess that when they are in the ecstasy of a sexual climax they are not aware of anything or anyone but the pleasure they are experiencing.

If you don't have the ideal husband, make the most of the situation and try to keep your sexual desires satisfied. Unrelieved desires that cannot be satisfied by solitary masturbation can lead to harmful tensions and dangerous triangles. The ideal man in your fantasies probably doesn't exist anyway. So don't give up a sure thing just to chase a dream.

### Satisfying Your Sexual Appetite

How often you have sex is up to you and your man. There is no recommended frequency that everyone can use as a guide. Surveys show that the average couple has intercourse about three times a week. When one partner desires daily sex and the other partner is a twice-a-week lover, the couple may have to compromise on four or five times a week. When a male partner insists on having sex more often than you desire it, there isn't any reason why you cannot oblige him as long as he does not insist that you reach a climax against your wishes. If you desire more sex than your man can supply in a conventional manner (remember that a man cannot attempt intercourse without an erection), your man's vanity should not be hurt if you ask him to relieve your tension occasionally with manual or oral techniques. Any man would experience pleasure seeing his woman enjoy an orgasm, even if he is only a spectator.

If your man develops an erection but is unable to reach a climax in intercourse, you may be able to masturbate him to orgasm. Remember that anything you choose to do together is perfectly acceptable.

### *There's More Pleasure in Moderation*

Be careful not to overdo it in seeking sexual pleasure. Frequent, *forced* sex may not provide the intense pleasure felt in more moderate sexual activity. Furthermore, sexual fatigue, though not physically harmful, may make it difficult for your man to develop an erection under any circumstances.

It's not unusual for some men to have difficulty maintaining an erection a day or two after being satisfied sexually. But a man who is consistently unable to maintain an erection during sexual intercourse usually has psychological problems that may require professional attention. If your man occasionally has trouble keeping an erection, don't criticize him or tease him about his problem. Fear of failure is one of the greatest causes of psychological impotence in men.

If you have a good, open, and honest relationship with your man, you can talk with him about any problems that either of you might have. You should be able to tell him what you like and ask for what you want. Getting the most out of sex with your man depends largely upon understanding and cooperation that will prevent a buildup of tension, fear, frustration, and resentment.

### How to Get Your Full Share of Pleasure

Although it's not a good idea to follow someone else's checklist in preparing for sexual intercourse (we're all different!), you should follow certain basic procedures in order to enhance the pleasure of making love. Kissing, caressing, genital rubbing, and other mutually stimulating activity, for example, will make penetration by your man easier and more pleasurable. You should do anything you and your man enjoy doing for as long as you want to do it, or at least until your genitals are well lubricated by your body's natural moisture. Some women become wet after only a few minutes of foreplay. Others may require prolonged foreplay.

### Be Active Rather than Passive

Once you begin sexual intercourse, you should be just as active as your man in your efforts to experience pleasure and to attain orgasm. If you don't thrust, roll your hips, and tilt your pelvis in order to get maximum clitoral stimulation, you may have difficulty reaching a climax before your man loses his erection. So try to use movement that makes good use of your man's movement. No matter how good a lover your partner may be, or how long he may be able to maintain an erection, it's up to you to utilize his presence and his movements to your best advantage. Your orgasm is primarily *your* responsibility. You have to *make* it happen yourself. Remember that any effort you make to satisfy yourself will automatically provide pleasure for your man.

## How to Calm a Quick Man

If you don't climax during intercourse because your man finishes too quickly, you can climax afterward with manual manipulation. Or you can repeat the intercourse later in the day—or the next day—when your man won't be too excited to maintain an erection for a longer period of time. A man who tends to ejaculate prematurely must often be calmed down by having an orgasm, with masturbation or intercourse, several hours before attempting to satisfy his woman with intercourse.

### How Roberta Calmed Marcus

Roberta and Marcus made love twice a week. Each time Marcus penetrated Roberta, however, he ejaculated within seconds. It was virtually impossible for Roberta to climax during intercourse, so she often masturbated during the day when she was alone. Marcus, who was ashamed of his failure and his lack of control, was often reluctant to approach Roberta. He was beginning to lose confidence in his masculinity.

Actually, Marcus was a sexually sensitive individual with a potentially large sexual capacity. When Roberta learned that Marcus might benefit from increased sexual activity, she immediately took the initiative and suggested daily sexual activity. It was only a matter of days before Marcus was able to prolong intercourse to three minutes or longer—long enough for Roberta to climax in his arms.

As long as Marcus and Roberta made love frequently, he had no problem with premature ejaculation. "The additional attention I have to give Marcus to keep him calmed is well worth the effort," Roberta confided with a wink. "It's also a good way to keep him home!"

## Advice for Beginners

If you are a virgin and you have never had sexual intercourse, you should not expect to experience an orgasm the first time you go to bed with a man. Some women experience pleasure the first time they are penetrated by a man, and some may even climax. As a general rule, however, the average woman must become accustomed to intercourse before she can enjoy it fully. So don't be disappointed if you don't "hear bells" during the early months of your first relationship with a man.

### Size Is Not Important

Inexperienced women who see an erect penis for the first time often fear that they won't be able to receive the organ without pain or injury. Actually, it is practically impossible for a man's penis to be too large to fit into a normal vagina. Every woman's vaginal tract is flexible enough to stretch in accommodating the largest male organ. If a vaginal tract can serve as a passageway for the birth of a child, it can certainly accommodate an erect male penis, which is tiny compared to the size of a baby's head. Besides, when you are adequately stimulated and lubricated, your vaginal muscles will actually distend in anticipation of penetration.

Contrary to the opinions of some men, the size of a man's penis, which may vary from four to eight inches in length, has very little to do with the amount of pleasure you'll experience. Since orgasm is triggered primarily by stimulation of the clitoris and the inner lips at the vaginal opening, a small penis may provide just as much stimulation as a large penis. An unusually large penis may cause a little discomfort during the initial penetration if you are not adequately prepared, but no harm will result.

### Vaginal Depth and Penis Length

Although the penis is fairly hard when it is fully erect, it is padded on the end by a soft, flexible head that prevents painful poking. The average vagina is only about four inches deep, but it lengthens easily to accommodate a penis that is several inches long. So don't worry about the length of your man's penis. Actually, the pressure exerted by the tip of the penis pushing back the uterus can be a pleasurable sensation.

If your man is knowledgeable and considerate, he will penetrate you slowly and cautiously to give you time to relax in receiving him. Most men now realize that it is better to be tender and loving than to display their manhood with fast and rough penetration.

*Note*: If penetration by a man proves to be difficult or painful, see a gynecologist for a pelvic examination. If there are no physical abnormalities, generous use of an artificial lubricant might be helpful. Surgical

K-Y jelly, available in any drug store, is a good sterile and water-soluble lubricant that can be easily washed away.

## Sexual Relief for Single Women

You've probably noticed that this chapter refers more to "your man" than to "your husband." The reason for this is that there are many women today who do not desire to get married and who choose to have a man without making any permanent commitments. Finding the right man for such an arrangement may be difficult, however.

If you are single, widowed, or divorced, and you are alone and sexually stimulated, there isn't any reason why you cannot relieve your sexual tension with masturbation. Contrary to popular belief, masturbation is not harmful. In fact, as a method of relieving tension, masturbation is a healthful practice.

Remember that a woman who can climax with masturbation is more likely to climax during intercourse than a woman who has never masturbated. So even if you are saving yourself for a special man, you should keep your sexual tensions relieved with masturbation until you find him.

### Technique for Female Masturbation

If you do resort to masturbation for relief of sexual tension, you don't need a phallic-shaped vibrator, a dildo, a set of Japanese Ben-wa balls, a finger extension, or any other commercial device. In fact, since a female orgasm depends primarily upon stimulation of the clitoris, you do not need a device to penetrate your vagina.

Since the clitoris is usually very sensitive, many women stimulate the clitoris by first stroking the tissues around it. This results in a gentle tugging on the clitoris, much like that experienced in intercourse. Then, as sensation becomes more pleasurable and orgasm approaches, the clitoris itself may be gently rubbed. (A small amount of artificial lubrication may permit more direct clitoral stimulation without uncomfortable irritation.) Experienced women often penetrate the upper part of their vagina with a finger in such a way that the clitoris is stimulated by movement of the hand or the finger.

Every woman develops her own technique and frequency of masturbating. Surveys indicate that a large majority of women masturbate an average of twice a week, with a frequency ranging from daily to monthly.

According to studies made by Masters and Johnson (*The Pleasure Bond*), some women are able to relieve menstrual cramps by masturbating! Contraction of the uterus and the vaginal muscles during an orgasm apparently helps relieve cramps caused by spasm of the uterus.

### Menopause Won't End Your Sex Life!

If you enjoy sex, you'll be glad to know that your menopause will *not* put an end to your sex life. Contrary to popular belief, the hormones you lose at menopause have nothing to do with your ability to enjoy sex. In fact, when you quit menstruating and you are freed from fears of becoming pregnant, chances are you'll experience an *increase* in sexual desire. As you grow older, your vaginal lubrication may diminish and your orgasms may be less intense, but you can continue to enjoy sex, even at an advanced age. Sexologists now maintain that you *never* get too old to enjoy sex!

Many elderly men and women give up sex simply because they feel that it is not nice for old people to make love. It is unfortunate that society seems to discourage sexual activity among the elderly. In addition to the pleasure provided by sex, there is now some evidence to indicate that sex and romance can actually improve the health of old people, so don't voluntarily give up an active sex life. No matter how old you may be, you should continue regular sexual activity, with or without a partner, if you desire to do so.

### Claudine's December Sex

Claudine had been a widow for 15 years when she married for the second time at the age of 60. "My sex life is just as good now as it was 20 years ago," she confided. "I've maintained my ability to enjoy sex by staying sexually active, but don't tell anyone I said that."

Congratulations, Claudine! And please forgive us for telling.

### *What to Do About Menopausal Vaginitis*

After menopause, some women develop a vaginal dryness that may make intercourse uncomfortable. If a lubricant does not prevent irritating friction, a gynecologist can prescribe vaginal estrogen creams that might be helpful.

## Keep Your Body Attractive

Your physical appearance can have much to do with how successful you are in sex. If your body is clean, trim, and attractive, for example, you'll attract more attention and get more response from your lover. Proper care of your body is as essential for a happy, successful sex life as for radiant health and beauty. So be sure to follow the complete program outlined in this book.

"Take care of your body," Mae West advises in her book *Sex Drive*, "and your body will be good to you." Although in her eighties, Miss West doesn't hesitate to admit that she still enjoys sex. She recommends "an organic apple a day and beautiful men as often as possible" for women who want to stay youthful.

## SUMMARY

1. Sexual love between a man and a woman should be a mutual undertaking in which both give and receive equally.

2. A female orgasm is more the result of clitoral stimulation than vaginal penetration.

3. Preliminary lovemaking erects the clitoris and lubricates the genitalia to facilitate orgasm during sexual intercourse.

4. Masturbation and other sexual techniques should be employed to relieve sexual tension when intercourse does not result in a sexual climax.

5. Every woman is capable of experiencing an orgasm!

6. Each woman must make an effort of her own to reach a sexual climax by utilizing the efforts and the presence of her man to her best possible advantage.

7. Virgin women have no reason to fear that they'll be "too small" or that their man will be "too big" to permit sexual intercourse.

8. Single women who do not have a partner for sexual activities should not hesitate to employ masturbation for relief of sexual tension.

9. Menopause should not in any way diminish your sexual desires or end your sex life.

10. No matter how old you are, you should remain sexually active as long as you have sexual desires.

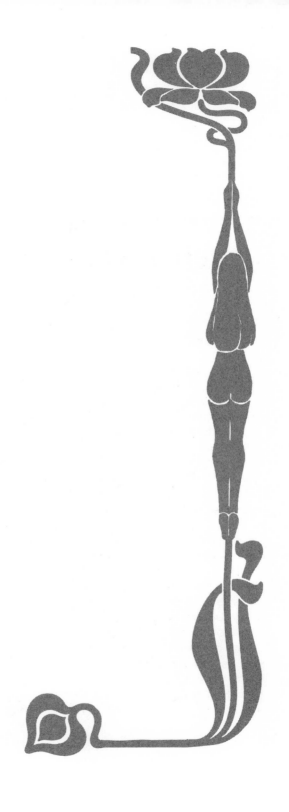

# *preparing for childbirth*

If there's any chance at all that you might become pregnant anytime in the future, you should begin preparing yourself for the occasion by eating properly and exercising regularly. You'll have a healthier baby if your body is strong and healthy, and you'll make a faster recovery from pregnancy. Well-developed abdominal muscles, for example, will aid delivery as well as protect against an abdominal hernia. We all know women who were unable to get rid of a potbelly after pregnancy. This is usually the result of stretching or rupture of weak abdominal muscles. Once this happens, it may be difficult or impossible to regain a firm, flat abdomen.

Long-standing nutritional deficiencies can deplete your vitamin and mineral reserves to such an extent that it may take many months to restore them, even with supplements. If you are deficient in calcium when you become pregnant, an increased need for calcium during pregnancy can result in loss of bone from around the roots of your teeth. This may eventually lead to periodontal disease and loss of teeth. Remember that your baby will take what it needs from your body. If you are already deficient, your body may be permanently damaged. Worse of all, your baby may not be as healthy as it should be. If you want to have a beautiful body as well as a beautiful baby, you shouldn't wait until after the baby has been delivered to begin an exercise and nutrition program. You should begin now! Remember that it takes time to strengthen a weak body and regain lost health. This should be done *before* you become pregnant.

184

# Chapter 11

## How Tina Won a Beauty Contest After Her Baby Was Born

Tina D. was an aspiring actress who planned to attract a little attention by participating in a state-wide beauty contest. Her plans were thwarted, however, when she became pregnant, but she did not give up. Two years later, she entered the contest and won! With the news clippings of her success as a beauty contest winner, she got a job doing television commercials. "I'm on my way," Tina announced with obvious confidence. "And I owe my start to my physical appearance."

How did Tina manage to have a baby and then win a beauty contest? She did it by following a diet-and-exercise plan similar to the one outlined in this book. Her body was just as beautiful after pregnancy as before. And with a beautiful baby and a loving husband, she continued to pursue her career.

Of course, not every woman wants to win a beauty contest or become an actress. But every woman can and should do as Tina did and make every possible effort to protect her health and her baby during pregnancy. How you care for yourself before and after your baby comes can make the difference between falling apart or staying beautiful. Some women who begin a health-and-exercise program for the first time during

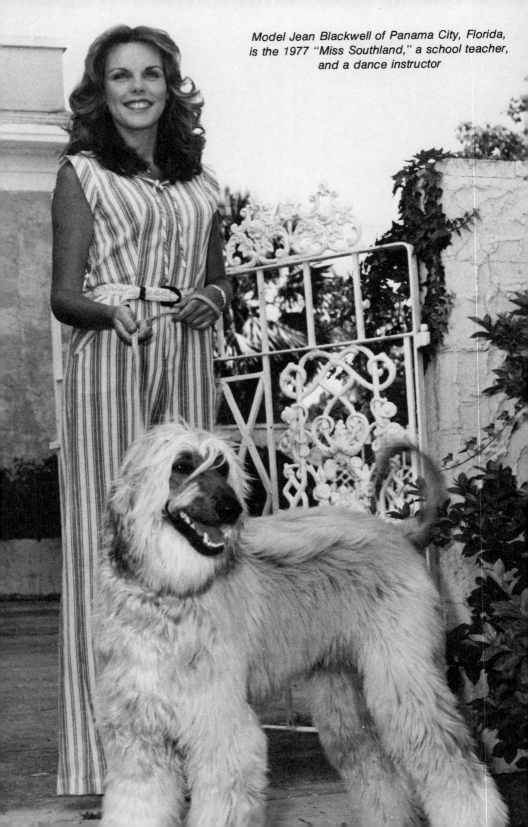

Model Jean Blackwell of Panama City, Florida, is the 1977 "Miss Southland," a school teacher, and a dance instructor pregnancy actually become *more* beautiful with continued use of the program. There's one thing for sure: If you don't make a special effort to eat properly and exercise regularly during pregnancy, you'll lose ground in your battle against aging.

## Good Nutrition Is Most Important

Good nutrition is essential in building a healthy baby and protecting your health during pregnancy. If you eat properly, as recommended in the previous chapters of this book, you may simply continue with the same eating program. It may be a good idea, however, to supplement your diet with calcium, vitamin D, iron, folic acid, and other vitamins and minerals to provide nutritional insurance for you and your baby.

### *How to Get the Nutrients You Need Without Getting Fat*

Doctors estimate that you will need at least 200 extra calories a day from the fourth to the ninth month of pregnancy, and about 1,000 additional calories a day during lactation. You'll also need increased amounts of protein, vitamins, and minerals. So you'll obviously have to eat more than usual. The only way that you can get more nutrients without taking in an excessive number of calories is to eat fresh, natural foods. You should eat *no* refined or processed foods. And you should avoid canned, packaged, or frozen foods whenever possible. Remember that there are many hidden calories in processed or packaged foods, and such foods are usually low in essential nutrients. You should *never* satisfy your appetite with foods containing sugar or white flour! You cannot afford to substitute empty calories for nourishing, natural foods when you are pregnant.

Make sure that your diet is balanced with lean meats, fish, poultry, fresh fruits and vegetables, and whole-grain products. Turn back to chapters 2 and 3 and study the material on diet carefully. If your doctor feels that you are gaining too much weight, you can limit your diet to low-fat natural foods. For example, you can get your protein from fish or poultry rather than from beef or pork. You can drink skimmed milk rather than whole milk, and so on, just as you would do on a natural foods reducing diet.

Many doctors now feel that a weight gain up to 30 pounds is not excessive if the diet is balanced with natural foods. Most doctors, however, feel that you should not gain more than 20 pounds. In any event, if you eat strictly *natural* foods, it's not likely that you'll gain too much weight, no matter how much you eat. And if your diet is balanced, chances are you'll get the nutrients that both you and your baby need. *It would be better to gain a little weight on a generous diet of natural foods than to risk toxemia or a nutritional deficiency on a restricted diet that includes refined or processed foods.*

### How to Use Supplements for Nutritional Insurance

When you are pregnant, it's always best to depend first upon *food* for the essential nutrients and then supplement your diet for nutritional insurance. You should make sure, for example, that you supply your body with at least 1,300 milligrams of calcium, 25 milligrams of iron, 8,000 units of vitamin A, 100 milligrams of vitamin C, and 400 units of vitamin D. It may be best to avoid taking extremely large doses of any single vitamin or mineral. An excessive amount of vitamin D, for example, may result in abnormal deposits of calcium in the body of your baby. Too much of one vitamin might create a deficiency in another vitamin, and so on. So, just to be safe, make sure that a balanced diet of natural foods supplies all the essential nutrients and then supplement your diet with at least the recommended allowance of vitamins and minerals. This way, the combined sources of nutrients, from foods and from supplements, will more than meet the needs of you and your baby.

Your doctor can prescribe a special prenatal vitamin-and-mineral supplement that contains a high level of iron, folic acid, and vitamin $B_{12}$. Folic acid is essential in preventing anemia during pregnancy, but it can be obtained in large amounts by prescription only. If a blood test reveals that you are anemic, you'll have to take more iron than the average woman. (Normally you lose from one to one and a half milligrams of iron a day, except during menustration when you lose about 20 milligrams. Only about 10 percent of the iron you consume is absorbed. When you are pregnant or menstruating heavily, you need considerably more iron than the recommended daily allowance of 18 milligrams.)

Remember that you should never try to depend solely upon supplements for isolated nutrients. There are many nutrients in fresh foods that are not present in supplements, and you must have these nutrients to absorb and utilize essential vitamins and minerals. For example, you should get at least 100 milligrams of vitamin C from fresh fruits if you are to get adequate amounts of associated nutrients that make vitamin C more effective. When you do take vitamin C, you should take it with orange juice whenever possible. So, no matter what kind of supplements you take, you must still have a balanced diet.

## How to Replace Missing Nutrients

If you're knowledgeable about nutrition (and you will be after you read this book), you'll be able to supplement your diet with the nutrients you need most. For example, if you're using skimmed milk and skimmed milk products on a low-fat diet because of a weight problem, you may need additional vitamin A. If you cannot tolerate fresh milk because of an inability to digest lactose or milk sugar, you can get your calcium from fermented milk products, which are low in lactose. If you don't use enough milk or milk products to equal one quart of milk each day, you should supplement your diet with at least 1,300 milligrams of calcium. (Remember that if you take calcium you should also take vitamin D so that you can utilize the calcium.)

If you don't eat liver, you may need additional iron and B vitamins. A newborn baby must have a high level of iron in his blood and in his liver to sustain him during the first few months of feeding on a low-iron milk diet. If you are deficient in iron, your baby may also be deficient. The iron stores of a healthy, breast-fed baby will usually last about six months. At the end of this time, it may be necessary to supplement breast milk with solid foods to prevent development of anemia. Bottle-fed babies are more likely to become anemic than breast-fed babies. So if you don't breast feed your baby, ask your pediatrician about early use of solid foods.

## Concentrated Food Substances Make the Best Supplements

One of the best ways to supplement a good diet with additional low-calorie nutrients is to use the natural food substances described in chapter 5. For example, you can get additional calcium from powdered skimmed milk or from bone meal, iron and B vitamins from desiccated liver, vitamins A and D from fish liver oil, vitamin E from wheat germ oil, and vitamin C from rose hip products. Brewer's yeast is a rich source of all the B vitamins, but it is so rich in phosphorus that it should probably be taken with calcium. You can get a phosphorus-free calcium in the form of calcium lactate or calcium gluconate.

## Avoid Poisonous and Artificial Products

When you are pregnant, you should not smoke cigarettes or take drugs or medicines not prescribed by your doctor. Nicotine and other harmful substances in your blood can harm an unborn baby or a nursing baby. Any artificial product may be potentially harmful to you and your baby. Try to avoid synthetic products as much as possible.

Remember that your nutritional requirements are *greater* during lactation than during pregnancy. If you breast feed your baby, be sure to continue eating properly *after* your baby is born. Go easy on the use of coffee and tea. The caffeine supplied by these beverages, transmitted through your milk, may make your baby nervous and hyperactive.

### *Watch for Toxemia!*

When toxemia occurs during pregnancy, there is a sudden weight gain with swelling of the face, hands, and feet, an increase in blood pressure, and a slowdown in kidney function. No one knows what causes toxemia, but some doctors feel that it won't occur if the diet contains adequate protein and other nutrients. If any of the symptoms of toxemia appear, see your doctor immediately.

### Special Exercises to Preserve Your Figure

Just as good nutrition is essential for preserving your health during pregnancy, regular exercise is important in regaining your figure following pregnancy. The best time to begin exercising is before or at the beginning of pregnancy, so that you can continue with the program through all nine months of the pregnancy. Then, when the baby is delivered, you can continue with the same exercises with only a few modifications.

Almost any kind of exercise will be okay if you begin early in your pregnancy and are used to it. You may even play tennis if you like. Just make sure that you start early enough to become accustomed to the exercise before you begin to feel the weight of your pregnancy. You should *never* start a new form of strenuous exercise late in pregnancy. More harm than good could result from unaccustomed exertion when your body is struggling to adapt to a rapid gain in weight.

No matter what type of exercise you normally do, there are certain special exercises you should do when you become pregnant. And you should do them along with any other type of exercise you might be doing. You can actually strengthen the muscles that you use in delivering your baby, and you can develop muscles that will preserve your figure as well as speed your recovery from pregnancy. There are at least four special exercises that you should do.

### 1. Wide-Stance Squat on Toes

Stand erect with your feet wide apart and *squat down on your toes.* Keep your back as vertical as possible. Hold onto a bedpost for balance if necessary. This exercise will stretch muscles and tendons as well as keep your hips and thighs strong and shapely. Try to do at least six squats each day. (See photo 1.)

If you begin doing squats at the beginning of your pregnancy, your legs will grow stronger as your weight increases. Then, after your baby is born, you'll feel as light on your feet as an acrobat. This is progressive resistance exercise at its best.

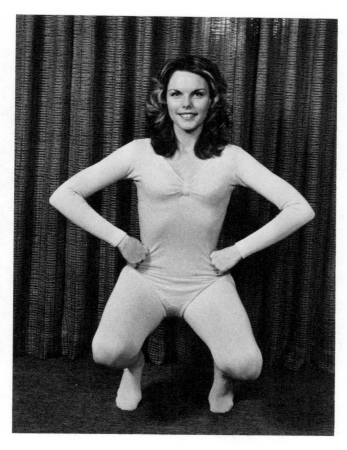

*Photo 1*
*The Wide-Stance Squat on Toes*

## 2. The Spinal Arching Exercise

Get down on your hands and knees. Arch your back up, contracting your abdominal muscles as tightly as you can. Then arch your back down until you look like a swaybacked horse. Exhale while you are arching up, and inhale while you are arching down. Arch up and down at least eight times. (See photo 2.)

*Note:* Regular bent-knee situps or trunk curls (described in chapter 8) will provide more effective exercise for your abdominal muscles during the early part of your pregnancy. But, when pregnancy becomes more advanced (after about five months), you can exercise your back and abdomen more comfortably by doing the back-arching exercise on your hands and knees.

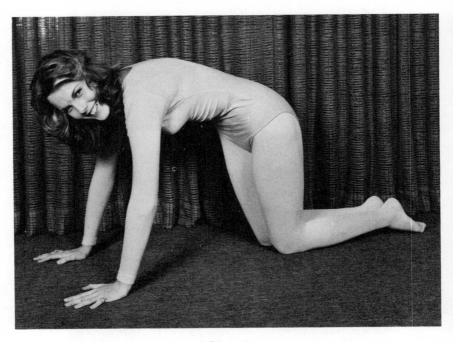

*Photo 2*
*The Spinal Arching Exercise*

## 3. The Isometric Breast Lift

Clasp your hands together at the level of your forehead, elbows pointed outward. Press your hands together to contract your chest muscles. (See photo 3.) Each time you press, there should be a visible lifting

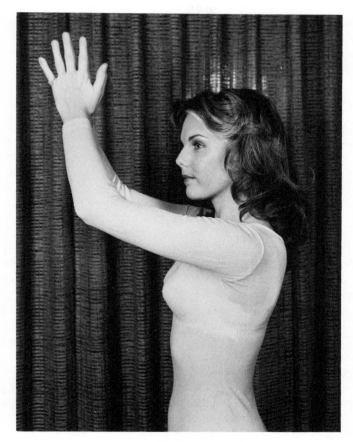

*Photo 3*
*The Isometric Breast Lift*

of your breasts. Repeat the exercise at least 10 times. (TV star Charo exercises her bust by pressing her hands together 500 times a day! See her photos in chapters 3 and 6.)

### 4. Pelvic Floor Contraction

Practice tightening your vaginal, anal, and urethral muscles by closing them as tightly as possible. If you'll simply concentrate on tightening or drawing up your anal muscles, you'll automatically contract your vaginal and urethral muscles.

Practice this exercise frequently during the day, before and after you have your baby. Once the muscles of your pelvic floor have been toned and strengthened, your vaginal opening will quickly return to normal after delivery, and your love life will be as good as ever.

### Balancing Rest and Exercise During Pregnancy

Although exercise is very important during pregnancy, it's also important to avoid excessive fatigue. So, while you should exercise more, you should also rest more. Make sure that you get adequate sleep each night. And, as your pregnancy progresses, get more rest during the day. Remember that the weight of the baby in your uterus tends to press down against the large blood vessels that pass through your pelvis. If this pressure is not relieved with frequent rest periods during the day, obstruction of the venous flow may result in hemorrhoids and varicose veins. Walking and other forms of exercise will aid the circulation of blood, but you should lie down periodically to relieve the pressure in your abdomen and your pelvis. The best way to do this is to *lie on your side* so that the weight of the baby will fall away from the large veins next to your spine. Lying on your back while you are pregnant can actually cause faintness (supine hypotension syndrome) by obstructing the flow of venous blood.

If you are a working woman, you should probably take a leave of absence from your job during the last three months of your pregnancy. Staying home will allow you to plan your day so that you can get adequate rest and exercise. If you are unable to quit working, try to at least make sure that your day is broken up with a couple of 10-minute rest periods every morning and every afternoon. Just lie down on your side and bend your knees and hips a little.

*Note*: A little swelling around your ankles may be an indication of interference with the return of venous blood from your legs, which means that you should lie down more often or elevate your legs. You should always bring swollen ankles to the attention of your doctor, however, so that he can watch for early signs of toxemia, high blood pressure, and water retention.

### What About Stretch Marks?

Once stretch marks appear, there isn't anything you can do to erase them. And they are sometimes unavoidable. If you eat fresh, natural foods to get the nutrients you need without gaining an excessive amount of weight, you probably won't develop any deep stretch marks. A little vitamin C will help keep your tissues strong and elastic so that the collagen or connective tissue in your skin won't easily tear or rupture.

Rubbing vegetable oil on your abdomen each day after your bath will help prevent stretch marks by keeping your skin moist and flexible. Some nutritionists maintain that rubbing vitamin E oil on the skin will erase as well as prevent the scars of stretch marks.

When stretch marks first begin to develop, they will appear as red, purplish lines. When healing is complete, however, these lines become silvery or grayish in color.

### Get Out of Bed as Soon as Possible!

After your baby is born, get back on your feet as soon as possible. If you're strong and healthy, you won't have to stay in bed more than a couple of days. You need plenty of rest, but you also need a little exercise. Remember that the longer you stay in bed, the flabbier your muscles will become and the longer it will take to regain your figure.

Begin doing your exercises as soon as your doctor gives you permission. With the exception of the squat, do all of the exercises described earlier, along with the following exercise.

### *The Bent-Knee Leg Lift*

Lie on your back with your legs flat on the floor. Lift one bent knee to your chest; then lower the leg to the floor and repeat with the other leg. (See photo 4.) Do several repetitions with each leg. Gradually work your way up to lifting both knees to your chest at the same time. After a few weeks, you may begin doing bent-knee situps.

It may be best to refrain from doing squats until there is no longer any discharge from your vaginal tract. After a couple of weeks when you do begin squatting, be sure to squat on your toes, keeping your back as vertical as possible so that no pressure will be placed on your swollen uterus. It takes about six weeks for the uterus to shrink back to its normal size.

Most women are fully active one month after pregnancy. But be sure to follow your doctor's instructions in the event you have suffered more damage than usual.

*Note:* You'll recover more rapidly from a natural childbirth, which does not require the use of drugs or anesthetics.

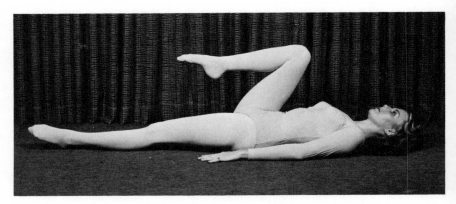

*Photo 4*
*The Bent-Knee Leg Lift*

### Breast Feeding Speeds Recovery from Pregnancy

It's always best to breast feed your baby whenever possible. In addition to providing your baby with essential nutrients and antibodies that will protect him from disease, *breast feeding may actually help preserve the shape of your breasts.* Some doctors, for example, feel that a breast that has functioned as nature intended retains its shape much longer than a breast that has not nursed a baby, and that there is less chance of breast cancer. Breasts are usually firmer and shapelier during lactation, but if they are very large it might be a good idea to support them with a maternity brassiere. Then, when breast feeding is discontinued, your breasts will return to their normal size without sagging.

Putting your baby to your breast immediately after birth will help your body expel the afterbirth by stimulating contraction of your uterus. *Breast feeding will also help reduce your bodyweight.* And as long as you are breast feeding, you probably won't begin menstruating until your baby is eight to 18 months old. Obviously, both you and your baby can benefit in many ways from breast feeding.

### *Sex, Pregnancy, and Lactation*

There's no reason to deprive yourself and your man of the pleasures of breast fondling while you are pregnant or lactating. No harm will result from handling the breasts. In fact, some doctors have noted that troublesome retracted or inverted nipples are seldom seen among women whose love life involves breast play.

Sexual intercourse (without deep penetration) is usually permitted up to the last month of pregnancy, often up to the last two or three weeks. Rather than risk infection that would require the use of antibiotics, however, it might be best to abstain from actual penetration during the last month. Penetration should *never* be forced when there is pain or discomfort.

In rare instances, certain chemicals in male seminal fluid can disturb pregnancy by triggering uterine contractions. Your own orgasm may also release a chemical (oxytocin) that can make your uterus contract. If you have a history of miscarriage, your doctor might advise you to refrain from sexual activity of any kind for a longer period of time than usual prior to delivery. Unrelieved sexual tension can, however, result in dreams that will trigger orgasm and uterine contractions. Generally, masturbation can be used safely for sexual relief (without penetration) during the last few weeks of pregnancy.

It will be necessary to abstain from sexual intercourse for at least two or three weeks following delivery. Ask your doctor when it will be safe for you to resume sexual activity.


### Megavitamin Therapy for Recovery from Illness

Just as proper nutrition, with emphasis on adequate amounts of the right vitamins, can help you to prepare your body for childbirth, so it can help you to recover quickly and thoroughly from illness.

In recent years, megavitamin therapy, or large doses of selected vitamins, has been used by some doctors and nutritionists in the treatment of illness. Although this method of treatment is still controversial, there is considerable evidence to indicate that it can be used safely and effectively in speeding recovery from a great variety of illnesses. Very little is known about the long-range effects of taking large doses of an isolated vitamin, however. So, while it might be beneficial to take megavitamins when you are ill or under stress, you should probably reduce your vitamin intake to a more moderate level when you are well again.

When you are healthy, simply making sure that you exceed your recommended daily allowance of vitamins and minerals will help prevent the development of illness. But when illness does develop, it may take large doses of certain vitamins to restore your body's reserves enough to recover from the illness.

Remember that there are many nutrients involved in combating illness. So no matter how many vitamins you take, you should continue eating fresh, natural foods in a balanced diet.

*Warning*: When you become ill, see your doctor for diagnosis and treatment. You may then use megavitamin therapy to make sure that your body has every possible advantage in waging its own war against the illness.

### How to Simplify Megavitamin Therapy

Every vitamin has a multitude of functions in the body. There are, however, certain basic needs in your body that must be met with certain essential vitamins. This allows you to simplify megavitamin therapy by taking a certain vitamin for a certain type of disorder. Any condition involving an infection, for example, may benefit from large doses of vitamins A and C. A circulatory problem might respond to massive doses of vitamin E. It is now well known that a high level of vitamin C in the blood combats infection and promotes healing, while vitamin E is a natural anticoagulant that prevents abnormal clotting of blood. Both vitamins C and E are antioxidants that help delay the aging process.

When beginning megavitamin therapy for the first time, always start with the lower dose and gradually work your way up to a larger dose over a period of several weeks. Discontinue large doses, however, if any ill effects occur. Be sure to study the material on vitamins in chapter 4 before experimenting with them.

### How Shawn Saved Her Marriage with Megavitamins

Shawn D. was desperately seeking help for an emotional illness that was threatening her marriage. Mental depression, irritability, and other symptoms of emotional instability were rapidly alienating her husband. "I'm constantly losing my temper," Shawn confessed, "and I take everything out on my poor husband. Sometimes he doesn't even come home when he leaves the office."

Chronic diarrhea, a skin condition, and an inflamed vaginal opening indicated that Shawn might be suffering from a vitamin B deficiency. She was instructed to take a vitamin supplement called "high B with C." Within weeks, her temperament and her emotional state improved. Her "incurable" skin condition cleared up completely!

"It's hard to believe that taking a few vitamins could change my mental attitude, but it's a fact that I'm a different person," Shawn reported. "I'm no longer irritable, and my husband and I are getting along fabulously well together." Shawn also experienced a surge of new-found energy. She literally bounced through a spring-cleaning program that converted her home from a "cluttered mess" to a neat, clean "model home."

If you are suffering from a vitamin-related disorder, chances are that you, too, will experience some obvious improvement after only a few weeks on megavitamin therapy. You should, however, continue with the therapy for at least two months.

### Megavitamin A for Skin Disorders and Infections

Vitamin A may be taken in daily divided doses ranging from 10,000 to 35,000 U.S.P. units for skin and eye problems and for chronic infection. Remember, however, that excessively large doses of vitamin A over a period of several months can have toxic effects. Too much vitamin A, for example, can cause skin problems that are similar to those caused by a vitamin A deficiency.

### Megavitamin B for Nervous and Mental Disorders

Vitamin B is best taken in a B-complex formula in which *all* of the B vitamins are taken together, unless, of course, your doctor prescribes a specific B vitamin for a specific disease or deficiency. Any high-potency B-complex supplement in which the potency of the various B vitamins ranges from 25 to 50 milligrams (or micrograms in the case of $B_{12}$) is adequate for beginning megavitamin therapy. Dosage may be gradually increased up to 100 milligrams or more.

High-potency B-complex vitamins are often used in the treatment of conditions in which there are nervous and mental symptoms. Some doctors use several thousand milligrams of niacin (or niacinamide) in the treatment of schizophrenia and other serious mental disorders.

If you want to take pantothenic acid and pyridoxine (vitamin $B_6$) for arthritis, take at least 100 milligrams of each along with vitamin B complex.

*Note:* Do not confuse milligrams with grams. A gram contains 1,000 milligrams.

Reduce your dosage of B vitamins if you experience heart palpitation.

### Megavitamin C for Quick Healing

Vitamin C is best known for its ability to speed healing and combat infection. A daily divided dose ranging from 500 to 4,000 milligrams is often recommended in the treatment of viral and bacterial infections such as colds and influenza. Vitamin C is also often prescribed to lower blood cholesterol and to neutralize toxins in the blood.

Taken in large doses, vitamin C, like vitamin B, must come from a combination of natural and synthetic ingredients. So, while you should strive to use natural vitamins in everyday health care, you may have to use some synthetic vitamins in megavitamin therapy.

Cut back on your dosage of vitamin C if you experience diarrhea or any other reaction.

### Megavitamin E for Circulatory Problems

Vitamin E complex is often used in the treatment of heart disease and circulatory problems. Varicose veins, phlebitis, and poor circulation in the legs, for example, can often be relieved, and clots prevented, by taking 200 to 800 or more units daily in divided doses.

Although vitamin E is a fat-soluble vitamin, no signs of toxicity have ever been observed from taking large doses. Just to be safe, however, you should probably not take more than 400 to 600 units over a long period of time.

*Warning*: If you have high blood pressure or a rheumatic heart, begin with only 100 units of vitamin E daily and then slowly increase the dosage monthly as permitted by an examining physician.

## SUMMARY

1. Good nutrition and regular exercise will assure a healthier baby and a faster recovery from pregnancy.

2. A generous diet of fresh, natural foods will provide adequate nutrients for you and your baby without building up excess body fat.

3. Lying down frequently during the last three months of your pregnancy will help prevent hemorrhoids and varicose veins caused by circulatory obstruction.

4. You may be able to prevent stretch marks during pregnancy by rubbing your abdomen with oil each day after a bath.

5. Get out of bed as soon as possible after delivering your baby and begin doing your exercises as soon as possible.

6. Breast feeding is good for you, your breasts, and your baby.

7. Smoking cigarettes, taking drugs, and eating artificial foods can harm a nursing baby as well as an unborn baby.

8. Large doses of certain vitamins may help speed your recovery from illness that is not related to pregnancy.

9. Always reduce the dosage in megavitamin therapy when ill effects are experienced.

10. See chapter 12 for tips on how to care for special problems with self-help methods that will improve your health and prolong your life.

# *everyday health habits to look and feel younger*

Practically everything you've learned from reading the previous chapters of this book will help prolong your life by improving your health. And if you put into practice what you have learned about caring for your body, you'll certainly look younger and feel younger.

In this chapter you'll learn about such common disorders as constipation, hardened arteries, hypoglycemia, and dowager's hump, all of which can make you feel old and look old. There's plenty that you can do to help yourself in the treatment and prevention of these disorders, and everything you do will preserve your beauty and your youthfulness for years to come.

At the end of this chapter you'll find a few tips on how to use vitamins in a special anti-aging formula.

### How to Eliminate Irregularity

People used to be reluctant to talk about constipation. There was occasionally some whispered reference to the subject of "irregularity." Today, however, with all the television advertising promoting the use of laxatives, there's just as much talk about constipation as about the common cold.

Actually, constipation is *more common* than the common cold, and it

# Chapter 12

may be more dangerous. You already know from reading the previous chapters of this book that slowed bowel function caused by a lack of adequate fiber in the diet may be a major cause of colon cancer. (Delay in emptying the lower bowel allows bacterial activity to convert bile acids into cancer-causing toxins.) The pressure of accumulating waste in the bowel can cause a variety of problems, ranging from headache to diverticulitis. Varicose veins may even develop in your legs as a result of circulatory interference in your pelvic area.

Although constipation is a hidden problem, it can obviously wreck a beauty and health program. It's difficult to be cheerful and vivacious when you are plagued by chronic constipation. Fortunately, there's plenty that you can do to prevent or relieve constipation. For example, if you eat properly and make sure that your diet contains adequate fiber and moisture, with none of the refined foods that breed harmful bacteria in your bowels, you'll eliminate a cause of constipation *and* colon cancer.

## How Often Is Enough?

Generally speaking, everyone should have a bowel movement at least once a day. It may be normal, however, for some people to have one only once every day or two. If you're accustomed to emptying your bowels every day and you are suddenly unable to do so for two or three days, you may consider yourself constipated. When you are truly constipated, your stool will be hard, lumpy, and difficult to pass.

Since we now know that the longer waste matter stays in the colon the greater the chances of developing colon cancer, you should do all you can to give your bowels every opportunity to function normally. One or two bowel movements a day will be best for most people. If your bowels don't move every day, but your stool is always moist and well-formed, you don't need to worry about constipation. Just to make sure that you don't delay the emptying of your bowels, however, you should follow the same daily procedure recommended for everyone else.

### Visit the Toilet at the Same Time Each Day

Probably the best time to go to the toilet is after breakfast and then maybe before dinner in the evening. It really does not matter *when* you go, however, as long as you go at the same time each day. You can actually *train* your bowels to empty on a regular schedule. Make sure that you go regularly, whether you feel the urge or not. Of course, you should never ignore an urge to empty your bowels, no matter when it occurs. Once you have conditioned your bowels to empty at a certain time each day, however, you'll rarely experience nature's call at times other than your regularly appointed time. This will be a great help in planning your days and your evenings without having to worry about developing a sudden, urgent, and unexpected need to go to the toilet.

### Don't Use Commercial Laxatives

Many people who are constipated because of a failure to visit the toilet regularly try to solve their problem by taking laxatives. Excessive use of laxatives, however, may only make matters worse by making the bowel dependent upon powerful, artificial stimulation. If you do use a laxative occasionally, remember this: When your bowels have been emptied by a laxative, it may take three or four days for enough waste to accumulate in the lower colon to trigger another bowel movement. So don't become impatient and take another laxative if you fail to have a bowel movement in a couple of days. Your bowels will eventually move again on their own if you eat properly and visit the toilet regularly each day.

*Note*: Don't use mineral oil laxatives! Mineral oil will wash oil-soluble vitamins from your intestinal tract. If you do need a mild laxative occasionally, or if you want to taper off harsher laxatives, try cascara sagrada tablets. This is a natural laxative made from tree bark.

### Eat Foods Rich in Cellulose, Bran, and Moisture

If you eat fresh, natural foods in a balanced diet, as recommended in chapter 2, you'll get enough dietary fiber to maintain normal bowel function. If you begin to have trouble with constipation, however, you may have to increase your intake of fresh fruits and raw vegetables in order to increase the amount of moisture-retaining cellulose in your bowels. You should also take a few teaspoons of bran with each meal. Be sure to drink plenty of water and juices to keep the fiber in your bowels soft and moist. Remember that if you resist or postpone an urge to empty your bowels, your body will absorb the moisture from the waste in your lower colon, leaving it dry, hard, and difficult to evacuate.

Dried fruits have a pronounced laxative effect on some people. Eat fresh and dried fruits at night so that you'll have a bowel movement in the morning. If you want a little additional help, drink something hot just as soon as you get out of bed. A solution made of dried prunes soaked overnight in hot water containing lemon juice and honey will work for most people.

### How to Take an Enema

Even when you eat properly and make regular visits to the toilet, there may be times when you'll become constipated anyway. Illness, a change in routine, emotional distress, and other disturbing influences can temporarily short-circuit the nerve impulses that regulate your bowels. This is usually nothing to worry about, however. If you persist in regular toilet visits, your bowels will eventually move.

Whenever your bowels fail to move after three or four days, and you begin to feel an uncomfortable pressure in your lower abdomen, it might be a good idea to take an enema. Too long a delay in emptying your bowels may allow fecal matter to become so dry and impacted that evacuation might be impossible without first breaking up the hardened mass with a probing finger.

Taking an enema is a highly personal procedure that you'll undoubtedly prefer to do alone. You can use a simple cleansing enema in the privacy of your bathroom.

Fill an enema bag with one quart of warm water. Suspend the bag on the wall about two feet above the floor. Lie down on the floor (on your left side if you're right-handed) and bend your right knee up toward your chest. Open the clamp on the rubber tubing and let a small amount of water run through to expel the air. Lubricate the enema tip and insert it three or four inches into your rectum. Let the water flow slowly from the enema bag into your colon by manipulating the clamp on the tube. Stop the flow of water when you begin to feel cramps. After you have received the entire quart of water, lie still for a few minutes to give the water time to penetrate and soften the accumulated waste. Make sure that the toilet is close by in event you cannot resist an urge to empty your bowels before you empty the enema bag.

*Caution*: You should not take enemas too often. Use them occasionally when constipation is becoming such a problem that you're considering using a laxative. When you're traveling or visiting friends and you need an enema, you can use a disposable enema kit, which can be purchased in any drug store.

Never strain to empty your bowels! In addition to causing or aggravating hemorrhoids, forceful elimination of a constipated or impacted colon may result in a painful tear or fissure at the bowel opening. It would be better to first soften the hardened waste by injecting oil or water into your rectum just before visiting the toilet. You can use an ordinary ear syringe or a disposable enema kit for this purpose.

### How to Save Yourself from the Aging Death of Hardened Arteries

Heart and vascular diseases are the nation's No. 1 killers, accounting for about 54 percent of all deaths. More than 700,000 Americans die each year from heart disease alone, primarily as a result of hardened and clogged arteries (arteriosclerosis and atherosclerosis). There are, of course, many factors involved in the development of arterial disease. Hereditary predisposition, sex, age, smoking, stress, high blood pressure, diabetes, overweight, inadequate exercise, nutritional deficiency, and the amount of cholesterol and triglycerides in your blood, for example, are all factors to be considered. The fact that you are a woman decreases your susceptibility to cardiovascular disease—at least until you reach menopause when your level of female hormones lessens. If your doctor tells you that you have an excessive amount of cholesterol or fat in your blood, however, you should make a special effort to reduce the amount of animal fat in your diet and avoid refined carbohydrates.

Most doctors consider blood cholesterol to be elevated when it is above 250 milligrams per 100 milliliters of blood, and triglycerides when they are above 150 milligrams percent. For radiant health and beauty, however, your cholesterol level should be below 180 and your triglycerides below 100. (Always ask your doctor to give you the results of any tests he has performed.)

Even if your cholesterol and triglycerides are at a normal level, a low-fat diet that does not include refined carbohydrates will be of value in preventing colon cancer and overweight. So, regardless of heredity and other unavoidable factors that might predispose you to heart disease, you can benefit from the dietary guidelines that are generally recommended to prevent hardened and clogged arteries.

### Go Easy on Cholesterol-Rich Foods

There is a great deal of controversy about the role of dietary cholesterol in the hardening and clogging of arteries. If your blood cholesterol is not elevated, you probably don't have to worry about the cholesterol content of fresh, natural foods that are low in fat.

Cholesterol is found exclusively in foods of animal origin. It is not a fat but it is associated with animal fat. If you trim away the fat from the meat you eat, drink skimmed milk and use skimmed milk products, go easy on the use of butter, and avoid fried foods, it's not likely that you'll get too much cholesterol from lean meats, eggs, liver, and other wholesome, low-fat foods. An egg or two a day in a balanced diet is a valuable source of high-quality protein and other nutrients. Liver, which is rarely eaten more often than a couple of times a week, is a good source of iron and vitamins $B_{12}$ and A. Both eggs and liver are fairly rich in cholesterol, but they also contain lecithin and unsaturated fat that help emulsify cholesterol.

### How to Balance Nutrients and Fat

There is some evidence to indicate that a diet deficient in certain B vitamins and other nutrients may be more responsible for abnormally high blood cholesterol than dietary indiscretion. Whether this is true or not, it's essential to make sure that your diet is balanced with all the essential nutrients. If tests reveal that your blood cholesterol is too high, you may have to reduce your intake of eggs, liver, and animal fat and increase your intake of foods rich in essential fatty acids and B vitamins. Since both cholesterol and saturated fat play equally prominent roles in the development of hardened and clogged arteries, both have to be reduced and balanced with soft or unsaturated fat.

Ideally, less than one-third of the fat in your diet should come from animal sources. The rest should come from vegetables and other sources of unsaturated fat. Remember, however, that fat should not supply more than 25 percent of the total number of calories in your diet. So, while you should try to balance the animal and vegetable fat in your diet, you should *reduce the total amount of fat in your diet*. Any kind of fat, animal or vegetable, is high in calories and can be fattening or harmful in excessive amounts.

Use vegetable oil in cooking and on raw salads. If you keep your intake of animal fat low, you won't need more than a few tablespoons of vegetable oil daily. Excessive use of vegetable oil might contribute to premature aging and a vitamin E deficiency. It might also contribute to the development of cancer.

Lecithin supplements are a good source of the B vitamins and essential fatty acids your body needs to combat a buildup of cholesterol and hard fat in your arteries. Supplements containing vitamin C, niacin, magnesium, choline, inositol, pyridoxine, and vitamin E are often recommended for lowering blood cholesterol.

### Triglycerides Are More Dangerous than Cholesterol

With all the talk about cholesterol, most of us tend to forget that elevated blood *triglycerides* also contribute to the development of cardiovascular disease. In fact, there are some doctors who believe that

---

#### three basic dietary rules

If you have too much cholesterol in your blood, include these basic rules in your dietary guide:

1. Get most of your protein from fish, poultry, skimmed milk, and skimmed milk products.
2. Eat plenty of fresh fruits and vegetables.
3. Do not cook with grease or oil, except occasionally with vegetable oil.

*Note*: Including a little bran in your diet to aid bowel function will help lower blood cholesterol by increasing the amount of bile eliminated through your bowels.

triglycerides and other forms of fat in the blood may be *more* dangerous than cholesterol. It is now well known that excessive use of sugar and refined carbohydrates is primarily responsible for abnormal increases in blood fat.

You already know from reading other chapters of this book that sugar and refined carbohydrates in the diet are largely responsible for over-weight, colon cancer, diabetes, hypoglycemia, and a host of other health-wrecking disorders. You have probably also noted that practical-ly all the diets recommended in this book, for conditions ranging from tooth decay to heart disease, are similar. This is because refined carbo-hydrates are a common denominator in the development of a great many diseases. This means that *everyone, ill or not, should avoid refined and processed foods and eat fresh, natural foods that are rich in fiber*. Follow-ing this one simple rule is the key to the prevention of many common diseases! So even if your blood triglycerides aren't elevated, you should cut down on your use of sugar and refined carbohydrates if you want to be healthy and beautiful.

### Do You Need Salt?

Excessive use of salt has been implicated in the development of hardened arteries and high blood pressure. Of course, you must have a certain amount of salt or sodium in your diet for good health. If you eat strictly natural foods, you'll probably get adequate sodium. You may even be able to use a little table salt safely, even while you are pregnant. But if you eat refined and processed foods that contain salt and sodium pre-servatives, and then routinely use table salt, chances are you'll get too much sodium. Use of salted, preserved, and processed foods is a double-barreled danger, increasing blood fat as well as blood pressure.

If you stick to fresh, natural foods, you'll be less likely to have high blood pressure or hardened arteries. Best of all, you'll be avoiding use of foods that have been artificially enriched with sodium and other danger-ous additives. The next time you pick up a packaged food, read the label. Chances are it will contain two or three sodium additives, such as monosodium glutamate or sodium benzoate.

When you have any of the symptoms of high blood pressure, hard-ened arteries, or toxemia, your doctor might advise you to eliminate the use of salt altogether. You can learn to enjoy the natural taste of the foods you eat. If you feel that you must use a seasoning to disguise the taste of certain foods, you can use a vegetable salt that does not contain sodium or you can use any of a variety of herbs and spices.

*Note:* The water you drink may be abnormally high in sodium. Ask your county health department for a water analysis. Artificially softened water is usually too high in sodium, and it may be low in the magnesium and other minerals you need to *prevent* heart disease.

## How to Cope with the Aging Fatigue of Hypoglycemia

Hypoglycemia, or low blood sugar, is a common cause of fatigue. It also accounts for a variety of other symptoms such as weakness, shakiness, depression, irritability, anxiety, and an inability to concentrate.

Generally, when your blood sugar is too low, you'll experience hunger, weakness, and trembling that is accompanied by a craving for sweets. Unfortunately, the more unusual symptoms of hypoglycemia are not often recognized by doctors, and those who are aware of the disorder often loosely blame it for all the symptoms of undiagnosed illnesses. The result is that the average woman rarely receives proper treatment for the vague and nonspecific symptoms of hypoglycemia. Most often she is given a prescription for tranquilizers.

### What Causes Hypoglycemia?

Most often, hypoglycemia is triggered by sugar and refined carbohydrates, which increase the amount of sugar or glucose in your blood. When your blood is frequently overloaded with glucose, your pancreas becomes so sensitive that it overreacts and secretes too much insulin when your blood sugar is suddenly elevated. The result is that so much sugar is removed from your blood that there is not enough left to supply your brain and your body with adequate fuel. Thus, while eating sugar and other refined carbohydrates will give you a temporary lift, an *insulin reaction* may drop your blood sugar to a very low level a few hours later. This results in a vicious cycle of seesawing blood sugar and a craving for sweets.

### A Simple Cure for Hypoglycemia

Fortunately, the cure for functional hypoglycemia is simple: *Avoid sugar and refined carbohydrates!* Rather than undergo a brutal five-hour glucose tolerance test for a positive diagnosis of hypoglycemia, you may first try relieving your symptoms with dietary measures. This would require eating the type of fresh, natural foods advocated throughout this book, with between-meal snacks of such high-protein foods as cottage cheese, baked chicken, skimmed milk, nuts, and so on. The *worst* thing you can do is to eat something containing sugar, as some doctors advocate.

Once your pancreas has been sensitized by the excessive use of sugar and refined carbohydrates, you must make a special effort to avoid them, or you may eventually become a diabetic. Your overworked pancreas will simply give up and stop secreting the insulin you need to utilize sugar.

*Note*: The caffeine in coffee, tea, and colas can also trigger hypoglycemia in susceptible persons by stimulating the adrenal glands, which in turn signal the release of stored sugar.

### How an Airline Hostess Corrected Her Blood Sugar Problem

As an airline hostess with instructions to smile perpetually, Bonnie T. was finding it increasingly more difficult to be pleasant and attentive on the job. "Sometimes I'm so weak-kneed, nervous, and confused that I can hardly carry out my duties," she complained. "My afternoon flight is pure torture."

A medical checkup by the company doctor resulted in a negative report and a prescription for tranquilizers. A diet questionnaire, however, revealed a probable cause for Bonnie's misery: functional hypoglycemia. It seems that in order to stay slim and trim, Bonnie had been eating only one complete meal a day, late in the evening before retiring. Except for a cup of coffee in the morning, she skipped breakfast. Then, at noon, she had her usual quick cup of coffee, a doughnut, and one scoop of ice cream. Within a few hours, she began to feel the strength draining from her body.

The solution to Bonnie's problem was simple, specific, and miraculously effective. She was instructed to pack a lunch of baked chicken, raw vegetables, and fresh fruit, with enough fruit left over for an afternoon snack. The results were immediate! Instead of forcing smiles and avoiding passengers, Bonnie aggressively pursued her duties. With a renewed spring in her step and a revived alertness, she looked forward to each new day.

As a result of the change in her eating habits, Bonnie ate *less* in the evening, so she was advised to eat something for breakfast to keep her blood sugar up until noon. By eating more frequently and limiting her diet to fresh, natural foods, she actually *decreased* her calorie intake, making it possible for her to *eat more* and still keep her body beautiful and firm.

There are undoubtedly thousands of women who have what they think is a nerve problem that could be handled better with nutritious food than with nerve pills. The type of diet that corrects hypoglycemia can be used safely by anyone and should be used by everyone. Don't wait until a problem develops to begin eating properly.

### Other Causes of Hypoglycemia

If any of the symptoms of hypoglycemia persist in spite of a good diet, be sure to see your doctor. There are certain organic diseases that can cause chronically low blood sugar. Emotional stress can also result in blood sugar problems by working your adrenal glands overtime. So, if you're having a bad time with your job, your home, or your man, it may be just as important to relieve your mental stress as it is to correct your diet.

Remember that your body's ability to handle sugar diminishes with age. You can get all the sugar your body needs from natural carbohydrates. Rather than risk all of the complications of diabetes late in life, it would be best to quit using sugar and refined carbohydrates.

### Gloria Swanson Doesn't Use Sugar

Movie star Gloria Swanson, who is still healthy and vivacious at the age of 78, refuses to use sugar in any form. "I won't even have it in my house, let alone in my body," she states emphatically. Both Miss Swanson and her husband, William Dufty, are actively campaigning against the use of sugar by promoting his book *Sugar Blues.*

At an age when most people are literally down and out, newly married Gloria Swanson is still going strong. She attributes her youthful verve to a sugar-free, additive-free diet of fresh, natural foods, supplemented with vitamin C and other essential nutrients.

### The Curse of the Dowager's Hump

Dowager's hump is so common among elderly women that many women think that it automatically accompanies aging. Not true! There's plenty you can do to prevent such a hump. And when a hump does begin to appear, you may be able to halt its development with supplements and special exercises.

Most dowager's humps appear after menopause when hormonal changes accelerate loss of calcium from bones. The calcium deficiency that allows soft vertebrae to collapse the spine into a hump, however, usually begins early in life, so be sure to study the material in chapter 4 on how to get adequate bone-building vitamins and minerals in your daily diet. And be sure to do the posture exercises described in chapter 8.

If you're already showing signs of a dowager's hump or a slumping spine, take the supplements recommended in this chapter and do the special exercise.

### How to Use Calcium to Prevent a Dowager's Hump

It takes a considerable amount of calcium to restore strength to soft-ened vertebrae. Just to make sure that you get enough calcium, purchase a supplement containing calcium, phosphorus, and vitamin D. Take enough of the tablets in daily divided doses with meals to supply about 1,000 milligrams of calcium a day. And, to get additional calcium with trace minerals, take *bone meal tablets* with meals to supply another 1,000 milligrams or so of calcium each day. (Make sure that the bone meal has been enriched with vitamin D.)

Don't worry about getting too much calcium. If you aren't taking an excessive amount of vitamin D, your body won't absorb more calcium than it can use. Any excess will be excreted by your bowels. Until your bones have adequately hardened, however, your doctor may prescribe additional vitamin D along with betaine hydrochloride tablets to aid absorption and utilization of calcium. Have an orthopedic specialist x-ray your spine periodically. If supplements do not halt the softening of your vertebrae, it may be necessary for your doctor to prescribe hormones.

Remember that you also need plenty of protein to rebuild your vertebrae, so be sure to eat properly.

*Note:* Arthritic calcium spurs are not affected by the calcium in your diet. Spurs are caused by bony irritation, and they will form even when your diet is deficient in calcium. Your body will simply take calcium from your bones to form spurs. Increasing the amount of calcium in your diet will *not* increase the size of the spurs.

If you suffer from kidney stones, check with your doctor before taking calcium with vitamin D. The type of stones you have will determine what type of diet you must follow. A deficiency in magnesium and vitamin B$_6$ has been implicated in the development of calcium oxalate stones.

### *A Special Exercise to Correct Dowager's Hump*

Do this exercise at least every other day. It is especially designed to use muscle contraction and lung expansion to prevent further slumping of your spine.

Place a small cushion on the floor. Lie down on the cushion so that it is placed directly under the center of the slump in your spine. Hold a can of beans in each hand at arm's length over your chest. Inhale deeply as you lower the cans back over your head to the floor. Exhale as you return the cans to starting position. Do 10 to 12 repetitions. Keep your arms straight throughout the exercise. (See the photo.)

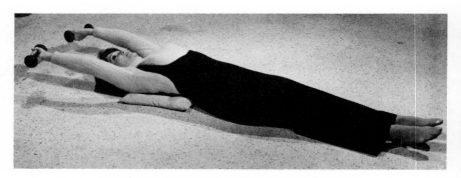

*The Straight-Arm Pullover for Dowager's Hump*

## A Simple Formula for Delaying the Aging Process

There are so many factors involved in aging, such as heredity, stress, living habits, nutrition, and so on, that it would be difficult to offer a simple formula for longevity. There is, however, much evidence to indicate that what you eat has a great deal to do with how long you live.

Dr. Linus Pauling, the 74-year-old Nobel Prize winner who wrote *Vitamin C and the Common Cold*, believes that good nutrition is a key factor in longevity. "I think that it is possible," he proposes, "that by proper intake of vitamins and other nutrients, and by refraining from smoking cigarettes and decreasing the amount of sugar ingested, life may be lengthened by 16 to 24 years."

Dr. Roger Williams, the discover of pantothenic acid (a B vitamin) and the author of *Nutrition Against Disease*, maintains that substances normally found in the body provide the key to good health and a long life. "If we use these effectively," he suggests, "we can cooperate with nature to prevent disease. . . . After 55 years in the field, I believe strongly that good nutrition is the key to expanding our physical, mental, and emotional powers."

### Vitamins That Prevent Premature Aging

A deficiency in any nutrient can accelerate aging, but there is considerable evidence to indicate that vitamins C and E can be used to slow the aging process or prevent premature aging. Both vitamins are antioxidants that protect essential fatty acids and cell membranes from destruction by oxygen.

Vitamin E gets the most attention as an anti-aging vitamin. Researchers have demonstrated conclusively, for example, that several hundred units of vitamin E daily prevents deterioration of blood cells exposed to oxygen.

*Using vitamin C to strengthen the collagen that holds tissue cells together and then using vitamin E to protect the cells from the aging effects of oxygen will improve health as well as help prevent premature aging.*

*Note*: After you have taken the anti-aging formula for three months, reduce your intake of vitamin A to 15,000 units, vitamin B to 20 milligrams, vitamin C to 500 milligrams, and vitamin E to 200 units. When you are healthy and your body reserves have been restored, smaller doses will be required to maintain saturation in your tissues. No one knows what long-range effects megavitamins might have on the body, so it might be a good idea to avoid habitual use of large doses of vitamins. During periods of stress or illness, however, increasing your intake of selected vitamins

---

anti-aging vitamin formula

Vitamin A—15,000 to 25,000 U.S.P. units in three daily divided doses.

Vitamin B complex—with 30 to 50 milligrams of each B vitamin once daily.

Vitamin C—1,000 to 2,000 milligrams daily in divided doses.

Vitamin E—200 to 400 units daily in divided doses.

(Begin with the smaller dose and work your way up to the larger dose over a period of one month.)

and minerals will help protect your body by maintaining or restoring reserves.

See chapter 5 for concentrated food sources of anti-aging nutrients.

### Observe These Precautions

If you suffer from gouty arthritis, a highly acid urine, or kidney stones of the urate or oxalate variety, check with your doctor before taking large doses of vitamin C (ascorbic acid). (Sodium ascorbate, a variety of synthetic vitamin C, may be used safely when the urine is abnormally acid. Persons with high blood pressure, however, should avoid use of sodium ascorbate.)

When you take large doses of vitamin C for a long period of time (during periods of illness), reduce the dosage gradually to avoid a rebound effect that might result in a sudden fall in the amount of vitamin C in your blood.

Remember that overdosing with one vitamin or mineral might create an imbalance in other nutrients. Too much of one B vitamin, for example, could result in a deficiency in other B vitamins.

Never take *large* doses of vitamin A or vitamin D for more than a few weeks at a time (see chapter 4).

### Health and State of Mind Determine Age

How much longer you have to live will be determined more by your health and your state of mind than by your age. If you are 70 years old, for example, and you are healthy and happy, you may have more years ahead of you than a 40-year-old woman who is in poor health. So forget about your age and concentrate on improving your health and staying beautiful. Think young and act young. Stay active physically, mentally, and sexually. Don't assume that you're old just because you've been on this earth a certain number of years. You may be much younger physiologically than you are chronologically.

#### Lauren Bacall's Secret of Youthfulness

Beautiful, green-eyed Lauren Bacall believes that "age is an attitude." Still young at the age of 52, she advises women to forget their age and stay active to stay alive. "Everybody should have work, or a hobby, that they can lose themselves in," she stated recently in a published interview. Bubbling with vitality, the busy screen star says that in many ways her life is "just beginning."

Why not make your personal health and beauty program your primary hobby?

## The Diseases of Old Age Can Be Prevented

Old age as we know it today is a *disease*. And practically all of the diseases that occur during old age could be prevented. If you eat properly, exercise regularly, and take good care of your body, you should be able to live to a ripe old age without suffering from the aging process. Best of all, you'll have a better chance of dying of old age rather than from cancer, heart disease, stroke, or some other disease, and you'll stay beautiful as long as you live.

## SUMMARY

1. Proper care of certain common, chronic ailments will make you feel younger as well as improve your health.

2. Regular toilet hours and a diet rich in fiber are essential in preventing and relieving constipation.

3. When your bowels fail to move normally for three or four days, it would be better to take an enema than to resort to laxatives.

4. A poor diet and nutritional deficiencies have more to do with the development of cardiovascular disease than any other factor.

5. Cutting down on animal fat and eliminating sugar and refined carbohydrates from your diet will help reduce high levels of cholesterol and triglycerides in your blood.

6. Go easy on the use of salt and avoid package foods that contain salt and sodium additives.

7. Hypoglycemia, or low blood sugar, can often be corrected by limiting your diet to fresh natural foods and by eating high-protein snacks between meals.

8. The dowager's hump seen among elderly women is most often the result of a calcium deficiency, which can be prevented.

9. Good nutrition is the key to preventing premature aging and eliminating the diseases of old age.

10. Your health and your state of mind provide a more accurate index of your age than your chronological years.

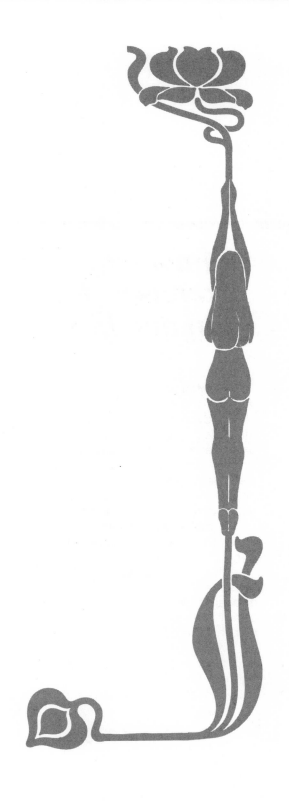

# slim-a-tonic and sex-a-tonic exercises for fun and health

Nothing is more aging than a broken-down body. If you want to look youthful and sexy, it's absolutely imperative that you take good care of your body. Almost without exception, women who are physically beautiful after middle age take some form of regular exercise. Take Doris Day, for example. She looks better now, at the age of 52, and has more sex appeal, than when she was younger! According to a *Family Circle* interview (September, 1976), it's her *body* that contributes most to her youthful appearance and her lasting sex appeal. "I constantly keep my body in shape with exercises," she says, "both isometric and conventional ones."

Remember that a firm and shapely body will make it possible for you to enhance your youthfulness and your sex appeal by dressing in a more appealing manner.

This chapter describes isometric and isotonic exercises that you can use to keep *your* body in shape. Use them regularly so that you'll be more appealing now and in the years to come. You don't have to have a specific reason for taking a little exercise. You can exercise for *fun*, and you can exercise to improve your sex life.

Many of the exercises described in this chapter have been demonstrated by Peter Lupus on such nationally televised shows as Dinah Shore's "Dinah's Place." You can now do them in your own bedroom, at your convenience, and at your own pace.

Have fun!

220

# Chapter 13

## Ten Slim-a-Tonic Exercises for Women*

These 10 iso-toning exercises are the best you'll find anywhere for a quick, easy tone-up of your muscles and a trim-down of your problem areas. Literally thousands of women who have followed the Peter Lupus program over the past 15 years have used these exercises with outstanding results.

Claudia H., a university physical education teacher, recommends the exercises for every woman. "You'll be delighted at the obvious personal rewards of Peter Lupus' exercises as your contours are reshaped when those sagging muscles become firm and tight. Use them regularly."

A South Carolina boutique manager confirms the proposal that these exercises are fun as well as effective. "These are the first exercises I've really enjoyed doing," she says. "Results were almost immediate on my waist and hips."

How long will it take to get results? Let Ruth Q., an Indianapolis bookkeeper, answer that for you. "I began to get

---

*Copyright 1975 by Peter Lupus, Jr.

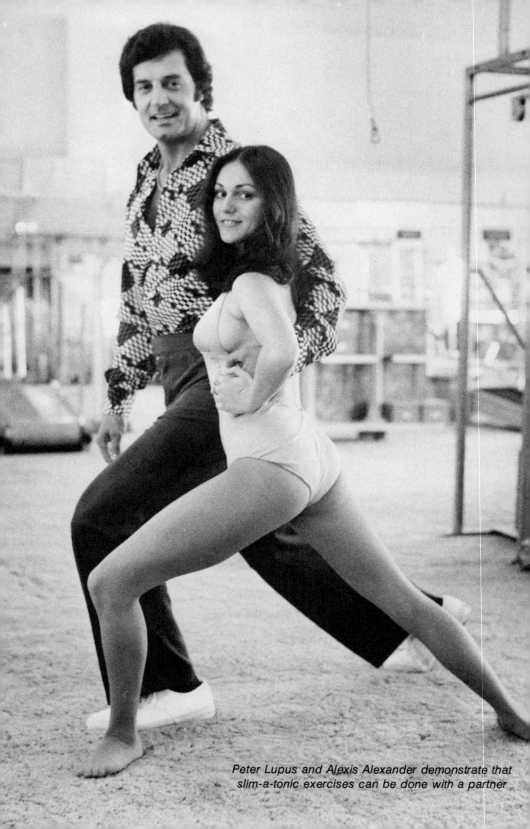

Peter Lupus and Alexis Alexander demonstrate that slim-a-tonic exercises can be done with a partner much firmer after the first week," she reported, "but I really saw results during the second week." She claimed she took inches off her waist, hips, and thighs in three weeks, along with an inch and a half bust improvement.

### How to Do Your Slim-a-Tonic Exercises

It would be best to do all 10 exercises every day. But if you prefer to concentrate only on one or two problem areas, you may do only the appropriate exercises.

Take it easy the first week or two. Don't strain too hard when you tense your muscles. To begin with, use only about two-thirds of your maximum capacity. And, unless you're already in good physical condition, do not hold a contraction for longer than a four count (four seconds) in any exercise during the first week. You may then increase the time to six seconds (six counts) the second week. As you become more fit, you may count to eight or 10 while holding an exercise position.

Don't get discouraged. These isometric-type exercises produce results quickly, as thousands of women have discovered. Some women respond slower than others, however, so please be patient. Do your exercises every day, week in, week out, holidays and weekends included. Even after you have achieved good results, you should continue with your program. Make your exercise a *habit* so that you'll *stay* in shape. All it takes is about one minute a day.

*Note:* In all of these exercises, count out loud so that you won't be able to hold your breath. Holding your breath during an exertion might result in dizziness or fainting.

### Exercise No. 1–For Hips, Buttocks, and Thighs

This exercise will reduce your hips, shape and firm your buttocks, and slim your thighs by smoothing and reducing cellulite areas.

Stand erect with your hands on your waist and your feet together. Lunge forward with your *left* foot, bending your left leg and fully extending your right leg behind you. Stay in this extended lunge position while slowly counting to three.

Return to starting position and repeat the exercise by putting your *right* foot forward. Hold for a slow three count.

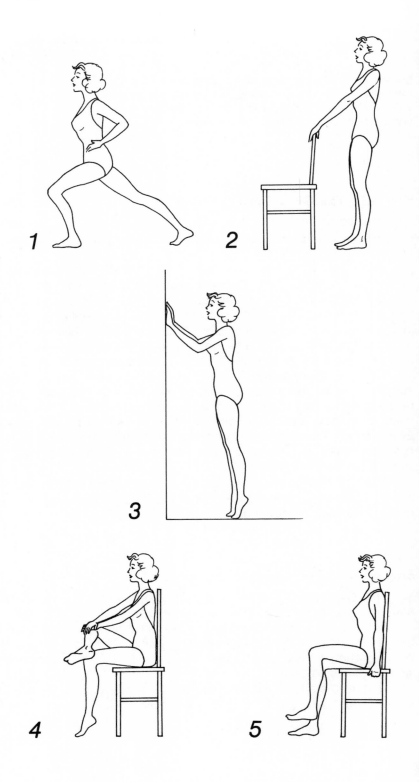

1

2

3

4

5

### Exercise No. 2–For Waistline

Use this exercise to firm up your stomach muscles and reduce your waistline.

Stand erect behind a straight chair with both hands on top of the chair back. Pull in your stomach muscles as far as you can and hold while you slowly count to six.

### Exercise No. 3–For Bust, Upper Arms, Thighs, Calves, and Ankles

This exercise will work your entire body, firming up and shaping often-neglected areas.

Stand facing a wall with your feet together and your arms extended straight forward so that both palms are flat against the wall. Lean toward the wall by letting your elbows bend. Rise up on your toes and push up against the wall as though you were trying to push the wall up from the floor. Push hard while you slowly count to six.

### Exercise No. 4–For Calves, Ankles, and Thighs

You can shape and tone your calves and thighs (and firm and reduce your ankles) while sitting in a kitchen chair!

Sit in a straight chair and cross your right leg over your left knee. Place both hands (one on top of the other) on top of your right knee. Push down firmly against your knee, resisting with your right thigh while holding your left heel high off the floor. Count slowly to three while maintaining the pressure.

Reverse the leg positions and repeat the exercise.

### Exercise No. 5–For Stomach

You can tone and tighten your abdominal muscles as well as trim your waistline with this simple chair exercise.

Sit erect in a straight chair and grasp the edges of the chair seat on each side. Lift your *left* foot off the floor and tense your abdominal muscles while you pull with your hands. Keep your muscles tense while you slowly count to three.

Return to starting position and repeat the exercise while lifting your *right* foot off the floor.

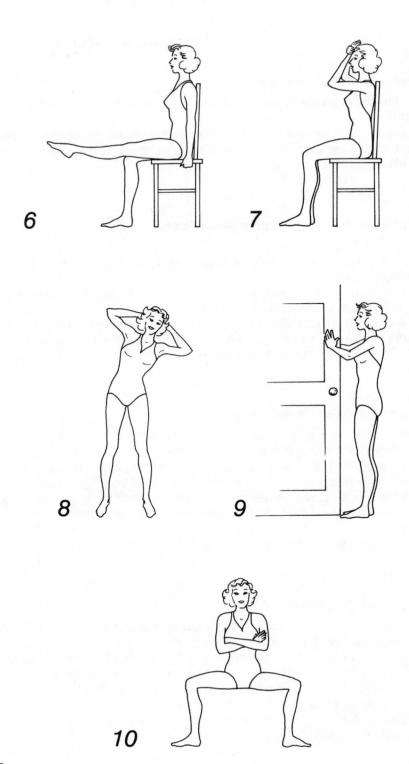

6

7

8

9

10

### Exercise No. 6–For Knees, Thighs, Calves, and Ankles

Put a finishing touch on a beautifully rounded thigh and calf with this easy-to-do, one-legged exercise.

Sit erect in a straight chair and grasp the edges of the chair seat on each side. Extend your *left* leg straight out in front, locking your knee and pointing your toes. Hold this position and tense the muscles of your thigh and calf while slowly counting to three.

Return to starting position and repeat the exercise with your *right* leg.

### Exercise No. 7–For Chin and Neck

Practice this exercise often to reduce and tone your chin and jaw line and to firm your neck area.

Sit erect in a straight chair. Place both hands (one on top of the other) on your forehead. Press against your forehead with your hands while resisting with your neck muscles. Maintain the pressure while you slowly count to six.

### Exercise No. 8–For Stomach and Waist

If you want to firm and tone your abdominal muscles as well as reduce your waistline, include this exercise in your workout.

Stand with your feet about 18 inches apart and your hands locked behind your head. Lean to the left as far as you can and hold that position while you slowly count to three. Then lean to your right and count to three.

*Note*: Be sure to keep your legs locked straight during this exercise.

### Exercise No. 9–For Bust and Upper Arms

Practically every woman is interested in toning, shaping, or developing her bust area. This exercise provides the best and the easiest way to do all of this.

Stand facing the edge of an open door. Place one hand on each side of the door at shoulder level. Squeeze the door by pressing your hands together until your chest muscles are tightly contracted. Keep squeezing while you slowly count to six.

### Exercise No. 10–For Hips, Thighs, Knees, and Buttocks

This unusual exercise will tone and reduce your hips, smooth and reduce the "waffle" areas of your thighs, and shape and reduce your knees and buttocks.

Stand with your feet two to three feet apart, toes pointed out. Cross your arms and squat down until your thighs are parallel to the floor. Hold this position while you slowly count to six.

### Ten Sex-a-Tonic Exercises for Women (Men, Too!)*

These exercises are designed to condition vital muscles in the buttock and stomach areas. By strengthening and toning these muscles, you can greatly improve your sexual ability.

If you like, you can alternate your sex-a-tonic exercises with your slim-a-tonic exercises, or you can do them all together when you reach top physical condition.

Keep these important points in mind when you begin your sex-a-tonic exercises:

1. For best results, have your partner do these exercises, too. Better yet, do them *with* your partner.
2. If you have any physical limitations, or if you have any difficulty doing these exercises, check with your doctor.
3. Go easy at first! Follow the instructions accompanying each exercise. Build up slowly to a full daily workout.
4. Warm up for each exercise by doing the first few repetitions slowly and carefully.
5. As with any exercise program, regular use is required for real results. So stick with your sex-a-tonic exercises day in and day out.

### *Exercise No. 11—Leg Crossover*

Stand with your back against a wall. Stretch your arms out on each side, with your hands on the wall for support. Keep your left leg as straight as possible and raise it forward and up to about waist level. Then swing your leg as far to the right as you can. Return to starting position and repeat four times.

Do the same exercise five times with your *right* leg, swinging it to the left.

---

*Copyright 1975 by Peter Lupus, Jr.

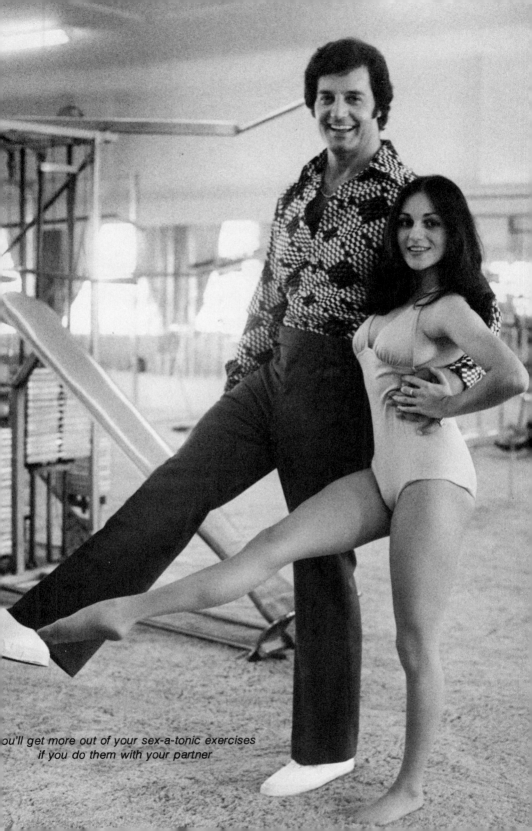
ou'll get more out of your sex-a-tonic exercises
if you do them with your partner

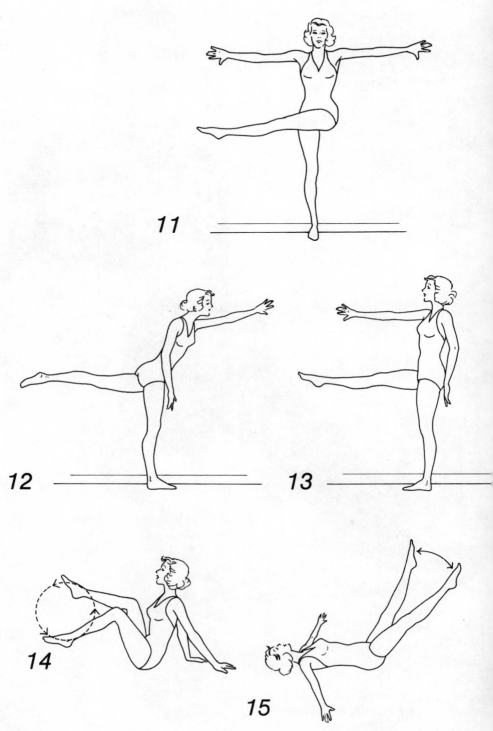

11

12

13

14

15

Increase the number of repetitions with each leg by one or two each week until you can do 15 repetitions with each leg.

### Exercise No. 12–Leg Lift to Rear

Stand with your left side to a wall. Place your outstretched left arm on the wall for support. Keep your right leg straight while raising it up behind you as high as you can. Return to starting position and repeat four times.

Turn around and place your *right* side against the wall. Repeat the exercise five times with your *left* leg.

Increase the number of repetitions with each leg by one or two each week until you can do 15 repetitions with each leg.

### Exercise No. 13–Leg Lift to Front

Stand with your right side to a wall, with your right arm on the wall for support. Raise one straight leg forward as high as you can. *Do five repetitions with each leg.*

Increase the number of repetitions by one or two each week until you can do 15 repetitions with each leg.

### Exercise No. 14–Leg Circles

Sit on the floor and lean back slightly with both hands on the floor for support. Lift both legs and rotate both feet in a circular bicycle-pedaling motion. Keep pedaling while you slowly count to five.

Increase the count by one or two each week until you are counting to 15.

### Exercise No. 15–Legs Up and Out

Lie on your back on the floor. Spread your arms out on each side, with your hands on the floor for support. Keep your legs straight and your feet together and raise your legs to a 45-degree angle. Hold them in that position and spread your legs apart to form a wide V. Return your legs to a closed position and lower them to the floor. Repeat three times.

Try to increase the number of repetitions you do by one or two each week until you can do 10 repetitions.

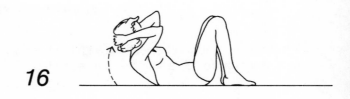

**16**

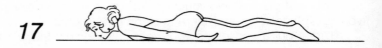

**17**

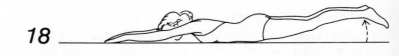

**18**

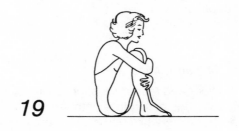

**19**

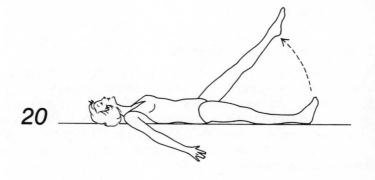

**20**

### Exercise Nò. 16–Quarter Situps

Lie on your back on the floor and lock your hands behind your head. Bring your knees to a bent position, with your feet flat on the floor and your heels close to your buttocks. Keep your legs in this position throughout the exercise. Curl your head and shoulders up from the floor about one-quarter toward sitting position. Return to starting position and repeat five times.

Increase the number of repetitions you do by two or three each week until you can do 20 repetitions.

### Exercise No. 17–Pelvic Tense

Lie face down on the floor. Tighten your buttock muscles and your stomach muscles simultaneously and hold for a slow five count. Relax and then repeat the exercise for another five count.

### Exercise No. 18–Rear Flex

Stretch out on the floor face down with your arms extended over your head. Raise both straight legs as high as you can. Return to starting position and repeat three times.

*Caution*: Take it slow and easy until your back becomes accustomed to this exercise.

Increase the number of repetitions you do by one or two each week until you can do 10 repetitions.

### Exercise No. 19–Situp Wrap-Around

Lie on your back on the floor. Rise to a sitting position and bring your knees up to your chest. Then wrap your arms around your legs and squeeze hard while tensing your stomach muscles. Return to starting position and repeat three times.

Increase the number of repetitions you do by one or two each week until you can do 10 repetitions.

### Exercise No. 20–Alternate Leg Raise

Lie on your back on the floor with your arms extended to either side for support. Raise one straight leg up to a 45-degree angle. Then lower the leg to the floor and repeat with the opposite leg. Keep alternating the legs until you have done a total of four repetitions with each leg.

Increase the number of repetitions you do by one or two each week until you can do 10 repetitions with each leg.

## SUMMARY

1. The exercises in this chapter have been perfected by Peter Lupus after 15 years as a consultant to the nation's top health spas.

2. For better health, a better figure, and a better sex life, make these exercises a part of your daily routine.

3. Do only a small amount of exercise to begin with and then progressively increase the amount of exercise you do over a period of several weeks.

4. You may alternate the slim-a-tonic and sex-a-tonic exercises until you are strong enough to do both.

5. Remember that regular exercise will lengthen your life as well as make you more physically attractive.

# how you can be a star every day of your life!

A wit once said, "Life is long and beauty fleeting." This implies that the good and beautiful things last only a short time in a life that is plagued by suffering. It doesn't have to be that way! Actually, life is *short*. It only *seems* long to persons who are in poor health. When your health is poor, beauty is fleeting. And each day may be difficult to endure.

When you are healthy, you'll stay beautiful, and life will be beautiful. You'll want to get the most out of each day. There isn't enough time in a hundred years to do all the things you'll want to do when you are healthy and happy. What you see and hear every minute of every day can be fascinating and beautiful. The taste of food can be delightful. Sex can be wonderful. Your relationship with your man can be deeply rewarding.

But for all this to happen, you must not let your senses be dulled by poor health or negative thoughts. You must devote as much time to the care of your body and your mind as you do to your job or your home. This means eating properly, exercising regularly, maintaining a tranquil mind, and taking good care of your skin, hair, and teeth. If you do all this, as you've been instructed to do throughout this book, your state of mind will be enhanced by good health and an attractive body.

Even if you aren't as physically attractive as Hollywood's glamorous stars, you can be a star at home. After following the programs outlined in this book, you'll know how to prepare healthful, wholesome foods for yourself and your family. You'll be physically beautiful because your body will be clean, healthy, and firm. Your skin, hair, and nails will glow with all

# Chapter 14

the natural beauty of an angel from heaven. Best of all, you'll know how to enjoy sex, and how to *increase* the pleasure of sex for yourself *and* your man.

With all this to offer, your man will look upon you as the most beautiful and the most desirable woman in the world. You'll be a star in *his* eyes, and that's what *really* counts.

## Mental Attitude Is Important

Your mental attitude is just as important as your health and your physical appearance when it comes to happiness. Remember that this book has been written especially for *you*. When the authors suggest ways to make you more appealing to your man, it's the self-satisfaction, the confidence, and the pleasure *you* get from your man's response that they are concerned about. So try to be a little selfish and keep your own welfare in mind. Strive to get your share of the happiness and the pleasures that life has to offer. It's important for your mental health that you do so. Unhappiness, frustration, and too few pleasures can lead to tension, pessimism, and depression. When this happens, you'll become a burden to yourself and to those who love you. It's difficult to find friends and experience love when you have a poor mental attitude.

Your attitude, good or bad, is contagious. If you're bubbling with happiness and confidence, you'll lift the spirits of everyone around you, and their mood will in turn give you a boost. But if you're angry or down in the mouth, this mood conveyed to your family and your friends will certainly increase your tension.

## Unrelieved Tension Is a Killer

In today's world, the modern woman is taking on increasingly more responsibility outside the home. More women than ever now have full-time careers. Some, many of whom are divorced, have the added responsibility of supporting children. The result is that more and more women are beginning to suffer from the same stress patterns that have so long plagued men. The stress of earning a living, supporting a family, and meeting the competition of opponents in the business and professional world is one of civilization's biggest killers. Unrelieved tension and uncontrolled stress can *wreck* your nervous system, resulting in a variety of physical and mental illnesses.

### Michael Learned: Modern Woman in a Modern World

Ask Michael Learned about the workload on modern women and she'll tell you that most women today work *harder* than women did in the past. In addition to playing the role of Olivia Walton on "The Waltons" television series, she cares for six teenaged boys at home! "I have more of a workload than Olivia," she says, referring to her TV characterization of a Depression-era mother of a large family.

How does this gorgeous-looking dream mother handle such a load in real life? By facing her problems and coping with them! She also has an established relaxation routine that she feels maintains a healthy mind as well as a healthy body. And, like most celebrities, she conditions her body for stress by eating properly. She has made a vow, for example, never to use sugar again. "I never put additional sugar or honey onto anything," she says.

Take a tip from successful women like Michael Learned and prepare both your mind and your body for your role in the modern world so that *you* will be able to cope with tension.

### Tension Can Be Relieved

There are many things you can do to relieve the physical effects of stress and tension. You should, of course, do all you can to reduce the amount of stress in your daily routine by controlling your activities and by maintaining a tranquil mind. But, if you have a lot of responsibility in your home or in your job, and the name of the game is stress and tension, you may have to do something each day to unwind in order to protect your health and your nervous system.

### Common Symptoms of Stress

Unrelieved tension caused by stress can result in a great variety of symptoms, such as a rapid heart rate, sweating palms, stomach cramps, recurring diarrhea, insomnia, and anxiety. Muscles may become in-flamed, causing soreness, spasms, and joint pain. If these symptoms are ignored and the tension isn't relieved, an overproduction of corticoid or adrenal hormones can lead to the development of organic disease. It is now well known that stress is as much a cause of disease as germs or a poor diet. Don't try to be a wonder woman and push your body to the limits of its endurance. Slow down. Relax. Relieve your tension, free your mind, and relax your body. It's essential that you do so to protect your health and your beauty. It's important to maintain a positive state of mind to be happy and to get along with people. If you don't, your attitude and your disposition will alienate your friends, your family, and your man.

### Beware of Mood Drugs

You should never depend upon mood drugs to relieve everyday tension or to calm your nerves. Except in cases of clinical depression, the use of drugs may do more harm than good. To get along in this world and stay healthy and beautiful, you *must* learn to cope with run-of-the-mill tension without using drugs. Don't take tranquilizers just because you think everyone else is taking them.

Sex is a great tranquilizer, but you have to be in the right mood to make love. Fortunately, there are some simple procedures that you can use anytime, anywhere, when you begin to feel tension gripping your body.

Lie on your back on the bed or on a thick carpet. Place your arms alongside your body.

*Step 1*: Beginning with the muscles of your face, wrinkle your forehead by lifting your eyebrows as high as you can. Hold this position of tension for about three seconds. Then relax your forehead and let the muscles of your face sag. Contract and relax your forehead several times until you feel that the muscles of your face are totally relaxed.

Try to keep your facial muscles relaxed while you relax the rest of your body.

*Step 2*: Lift your forearms and hands several inches off the floor by bending only your elbows. Hold your elbows in a partially bent position for about three seconds. Then let your arms fall back to the floor. If you relax adequately, your arms should drop like a rock.

Until you do learn how to relax, you may find it difficult to relax your muscles enough to drop your arms without assisting with muscle tension. Lift and drop your forearms several times until your arms are loose and relaxed.

*Step 3*: Finally, while keeping the muscles of your face and arms relaxed, begin relaxing your legs. With your heels about 12 inches apart, turn your feet inward so that you touch your big toes together. Hold this position of tension for about three seconds and then suddenly relax so that your feet flop apart. Repeat several times. Concentrate on *total relaxation* so that your feet and legs will be lifeless when you release the tension. (See the figure.)

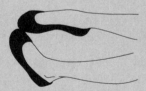

*Hold your feet in this position for three seconds before releasing the tension*

Remember to keep *all* of your muscles relaxed while you are relaxing your legs.

When you have succeeded in relaxing your muscles, try to be as limp as a dishrag while you lie on the floor. Concentrate on keeping your facial muscles relaxed. (Generally, if you can erase facial tension, your other muscles will also relax.) Imagine that you are lying on a deserted beach that is being caressed by a gentle surf and a soft breeze. Erase all cares and concerns from your mind. If you succeed in relaxing completely, you'll get up refreshed and your mind will be calm and clear.

## How to Use Your Mind to Relax Your Muscles

Many people do not know how to relax, and some people *never* relax. Chronic tension can become such a habit that the afflicted individuals walk around with their neck muscles contracted, their jaws clenched, and their hands balled up into fists. And when these unfortunate individuals sleep, their muscles *stay* tense. Most of them do not even realize that they are tense. They simply cannot distinguish between being tense and being relaxed.

Use the exercises on the facing page to *make* your muscles relax and to help you learn how to *stay* relaxed. Do them at a time when you know you won't be disturbed.

## How to Rub Away Tension

Everybody loves a body massage! When your muscles are tired, sore, and fatigued from chronic tension, special circulatory massage will flush out waste products and relax your body with a fresh flow of warm blood. Self-massage is simple. All you need is a little oil, cream, or cocoa butter. Professional masseurs and masseuses often use a mixture of min-

---

massage

*Beginning with your legs* (in a sitting position), rub from your ankle to your knee. Use long, stroking movements with your fingertips and the palms of your hands. You can cover your entire lower leg with one stroke if you place one hand on each side of your leg. Repeat at least three times. Then stroke from your knee to your hip, covering all sides of your thigh.

*To massage your abdomen*, lie on your back and stroke your abdomen from your pelvis to your breasts. Knead deeply but not so heavily that discomfort results. Place both hands side by side so that you cover your entire abdomen in one stroke. Repeat at least three times.

*Massage your arms* while you are still lying on your back. Extend one arm over your chest and rub it from your wrist to your shoulder in one long, stroking movement. Stroke both sides of each arm at least three times.

For additional circulatory stimulation, rub the oil off your body with a cold, damp towel, or simply take a cool shower followed by a brisk towel rub.

eral oil and alcohol. Evaporation of the alcohol prevents a buildup of excess oil. Use as much oil as necessary, however, to reduce comfortable friction and to make massage smooth and easy.

All you have to do is put a little oil on your hands and rub the large muscles of your body. Always start at the far end of the muscle and *rub toward your heart.* This will aid the flow of return venous blood so that your muscles can be flushed with a fresh flow of blood.

It goes without saying that the best way to get an overall body massage is to have someone do it for you. This will make it possible to get a delicious back massage. Why not have your man give you a full, nude body massage? And why not finish the massage by having sex? Making love while your body is oiled and stimulated following a massage can be a delightful new experience.

### How to Relieve Tension and Soreness with Moist Heat

Application of moist heat is a good way to relieve tension when you want a good night's sleep. For isolated muscle tension or soreness, all you have to do is lay a hot-water bottle or an insulated heating pad on a damp towel that has been placed directly over the involved muscles.

For *total* body relaxation, fill a tub with warm water and soak in the water for at least 10 minutes. Adjust the inflow and the overflow so that the temperature of the water will stay comfortably warm. Remember that water that is too hot (or too cold) will be stimulating rather than relaxing.

### How to Combat Tension with Supplements

There's no longer any doubt that persons under great stress can benefit from special food supplements. It is now well known, for example, that stress burns large amounts of vitamin C in the production of adrenalin. Most of the B vitamins are involved in the metabolic processes that produce energy. Such minerals as calcium and magnesium are essential in the control of tension in nerves and muscles. A deficiency in the trace mineral chromium has been found to be involved in blood sugar problems. There are many nutrients involved in withstanding stress, and the only way you can be assured of getting *all* of these nutrients is to eat fresh, natural foods in a balanced diet. When stress and tension become pronounced, however, it would be a good idea to supplement your diet with certain tension-fighting nutrients to protect your health.

*B with C Is Most Important*

A deficiency in any B vitamin can be a factor in nervousness and fatigue resulting from stress. Since *all* of the B vitamins work together, you should take *vitamin B complex* to strengthen your nerves. Brewer's yeast, desiccated liver, and wheat germ are the best natural sources of B vitamins.

Since vitamin C is also important in withstanding stress, many B-complex formulas now include vitamin C. Try to make sure that you get at least 1,000 milligrams of vitamin C daily when you are under great stress.

*Note*: Remember that taking birth control pills contributes to a deficiency in B vitamins, especially vitamin B6 (pyridoxine). Take *high-potency* vitamin B complex if you use the pill.

*Nature's Tranquilizers*

Calcium and magnesium have been labeled "natural tranquilizers" by some nutritionists. A deficiency in either of these minerals can result in a variety of nervous symptoms. Dolomite, or powdered limestone, is rich in both calcium and magnesium and is often recommended for unsteady nerves. (The recommended daily allowance for magnesium is 400 milligrams, and for calcium 1,000 milligrams.)

*Tryptophane*—something new! We've all heard people say that a glass of warm milk at night will relax nerves and muscles and induce sleep. Until recently, nutritionists thought that it was the calcium in the milk that did the job. Now it's believed that it is tryptophane, a protein substance, that lulls the brain to sleep. Some doctors now prescribe tryptophane along with B-complex vitamins to relieve nervousness and aid sleep.

## SUMMARY

1. When you are healthy, life is more interesting and you'll attract more attention from your man.

2. Your state of mind has much to do with how you feel and how people feel about you.

3. Uncontrolled stress and unrelieved tension can have damaging effects on your body and your mind.

4. Simple techniques used to relax your muscles can have a rejuvenating effect on your nervous system.

5. The circulatory-massage techniques described in this chapter can be used to flush out the waste products of chronic tension.

6. Moist heat is the most effective treatment available for relaxing tight, sore muscles.

7. Persons under stress need extra vitamin B complex, vitamin C, calcium, magnesium, and other vitamins and minerals to maintain a healthy nervous system.

8. Women who take birth control pills tend to be deficient in the B vitamins they need to combat depression.

9. Be sure to give your body, mind, and nervous system equal attention in your daily health program.

10. Remember that a good relationship with your man depends as much upon your mental attitude as upon your health.

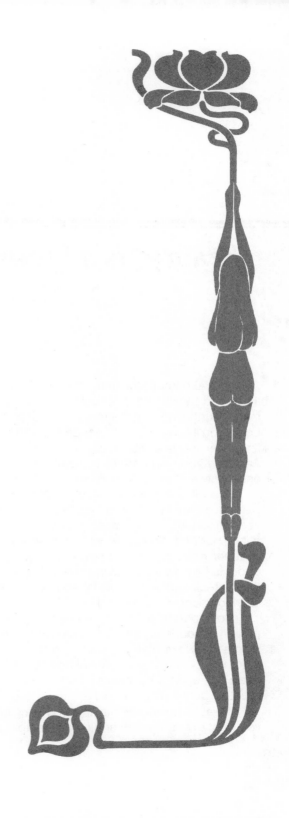

# beauty is a lifetime reward

You already know from reading the previous chapters of this book that good health is a prerequisite for happiness in old age. If you're still fairly young and you permanently adopt the programs outlined in this book, you'll have a good chance of living a long, healthy, and happy life. It's never too late, however, to undertake a self-improvement program. And how you take care of yourself from day to day can make the difference between living and dying, literally and figuratively.

Even if you are healthy, your state of mind and your daily activities can have much to do with how happy you are and how long you live. It's very important, for example, that you maintain an active and optimistic mind. *Hobbies and other activities should be employed to satisfy your inherent need to accomplish something constructive each day.* Dinah Shore is fully aware of the importance of achievement after middle age. "I think a feeling of achievement and being loved makes a *big* difference in staying young," she says.

Your personal health-and-beauty program should occupy a good portion of your daily activity. There isn't a better or more rewarding hobby than a daily exercise program and the study of nutrition. You can enjoy food, love, and achievement at any age if you pay your dues in personal health care. Staying healthy and beautiful at an advanced age is the greatest achievement of all!

It's absolutely essential that you stay active physically and mentally if you want to stay healthy and delay the aging process. Do as Jane Russell

# Chapter 15

does and develop new interests so that you'll never be at a loss for an interesting, constructive hobby. "I'll never stop doing something," she maintains. "If it isn't acting, it will be decorating, painting, designing, or building. I'll never be idle." Now 54 years of age, Miss Russell is presently writing her autobiography. This beautiful, intelligent woman is not content to rest upon her success as an internationally famous movie actress. She is too busy preparing for the future! Her mother, 86-year-old Geraldine Russell, is still conducting religious services in her backyard chapel.

Make sure that you, too, prepare for the future so that you won't be idle. Dr. Frank Caprio, the author of *Add Life to Your Years*,* advises that enjoyment of life in later years is an *art*. "It requires careful, systematic planning well in advance," he writes. "With advancing years this planning grows increasingly important. If you are resolved to live a long time, you should make some effort to get as much out of your added years as is humanly possible."

Dr. Caprio, a 70-year-old retired psychiatrist, is the author of 28 books and is still writing. (He is also the author of the foreword of this book.) Follow his advice and strive to make your retirement years the best years of your life. Adopt the health-and-beauty program outlined in this book and start making plans *now* for a long, interesting, and useful life!

---

*Citadel Press, Secaucus, New Jersey, 1975.

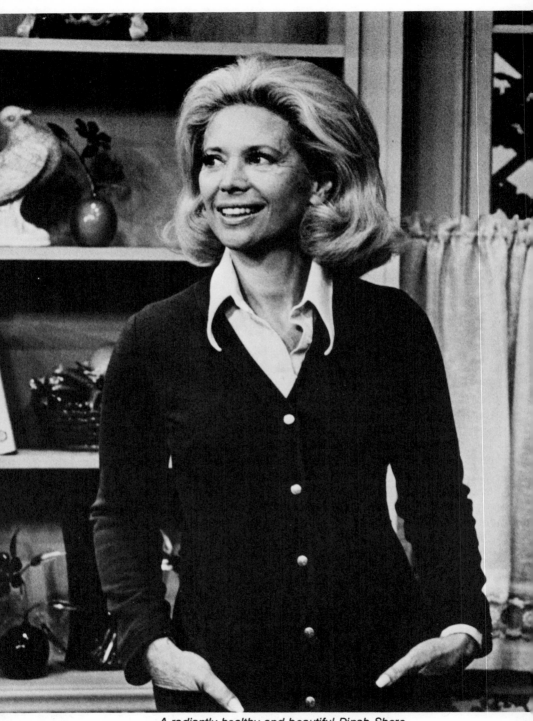

*A radiantly healthy and beautiful Dinah Shore
hosts the highly successful CBS-TV show "Dinah"*

## SUMMARY

1. You'll get out of your retirement years what you put into them.

2. If you don't take good care of your health, stay active physically and mentally, and plan for the future, your declining years will be burdened by poor health, boredom, and unhappiness.

3. If you follow the programs outlined in this book, you'll be preparing for the future that begins *today*!

4. Try to adopt satisfying hobbies that provide a sense of accomplishment.

5. Your personal health and beauty program can be a rewarding lifetime hobby.

# *Index*